The
HEALER'S MANUAL

About the Author

Ted Andrews was a full-time author, student, and teacher in the metaphysical and spiritual fields. He conducted seminars, symposiums, workshops, and lectures throughout the country on many facets of ancient mysticism. Ted worked with past-life analysis, auric interpretation, numerology, the tarot, and the Qabala as methods of developing and enhancing inner potential. He was a clairvoyant and certified in spiritual mediumship, basic hypnosis, and acupressure. Ted was also involved in the study and use of herbs as an alternative path. In addition to writing several books, he was a contributing author to various metaphysical magazines. He passed away in 2009.

THE
HEALER'S MANUAL

*A Beginner's Guide to Energy Healing
for Yourself and Others*

TED ANDREWS

Llewellyn Publications
Woodbury, Minnesota

REVISED EDITION
Sixth Printing, 2012

First edition, twelve printings

Book design and layout by Joanna Willis
Cover design by Lisa Novak
Cover image © ImageZoo
Editing by Tom Bilstad
Interior illustrations by Llewellyn art department on pages 54–55, 87, 155, 170–171, 193, 200
Interior illustrations by Mary Ann Zapalac on pages 46, 48, 50, 52–53, 71, 73, 77, 83, 90–103, 108–109, 135, 137, 141–142, 151, 192, 201, 235–236

Llewellyn is a registered trademark of Llewellyn Worldwide Ltd.

The Cataloging-in-Publication Data for *The Healer's Manual* **is on file at the Library of Congress.**

ISBN 13: 978-0-87542-007-3
ISBN 10: 0-87542-007-9

Llewellyn Publications
A Division of Llewellyn Worldwide Ltd.
2143 Wooddale Drive
Woodbury, MN 55125-2989
www.llewellyn.com

Printed in the United States of America

Other Books by Ted Andrews

Animal Speak

Crystal Balls & Crystal Bowls

Dream Alchemy

Enchantment of the Faerie Realm

How to Develop and Use Psychic Touch

How to Heal with Color

How to Meet and Work with Spirit Guides

How to See and Read the Aura

How to Uncover Your Past Lives

Imagick

Magical Dance

Sacred Sounds

The Sacred Power in Your Name

Simplified Qabala Magick

To St. E's second shift I.C.U., past and present.

CONTENTS

Part 5: Vibrational Healing Through the Sense of Taste

Part 6: Vibrational Healing Through the Sense of Smell

introduction

"PHYSICIAN, HEAL THYSELF"

A nyone can heal. Anyone can learn to administer energies that accelerate and facilitate the healing process. This can be done physically, emotionally, mentally, and spiritually.

The human essence is a wondrous thing! Its capacity to rejuvenate and regenerate itself is limited solely by our awareness. The amount of energy available to each of us to manifest and impact upon our lives—physically and spiritually—is limited solely by our capacity to give birth to greater love to ourselves and to others.

There currently exist many methods of healing and doctoring. Everyone you speak to has a different perception as to which is best. The truth is that the only one that is best is the one that works for you. Each of us is unique. We each have our own individual energy system, and to generalize and lump all symptoms, problems, and their respective causes and cures into one category does a great disservice to us.

Part of our responsibility as an individual, creative human being is to find that method or combination of methods that work best for us as individuals. This involves time and study—something many are unwilling to do in our present society. It always surprises me how generally ignorant people are of their own bodies and how they function.

In the past most people have given over that responsibility of self-knowledge to others, such as our medical doctors. Doctors are not gods. They may know more about the human body in general than most individuals, but nobody knows more about your own individual body than you. Unfortunately, few acknowledge this or pay attention to the intimate signals that their bodies send to them. We have reached a point in society (due to rising medical costs, etc.) where there is a need to take greater responsibility for the care of our own bodies back upon ourselves.

Above the portals of the ancient mystery schools—those higher centers of learning, healing, and spirituality—were but two words: "Know thyself"! The key to all learning, all balance in all areas of our life, lies within that precept. "Know thyself"—a simple enough axiom—and yet it is one that creates tremendous difficulty for many. Most people are unwilling to take the time to know themselves, and thus they give that responsibility and that power over to others. They hire others to know for them. This is comparable to having someone eat for you, go to the bathroom for you, etc. Theoretically, it sounds good, but ultimately it cannot be done.

All healing comes from within. The body has a tremendous capacity for restoring itself to health. Yes, because of genetics and such things as karma, there can be a greater predisposition or susceptibility to certain kinds of problems. Orthodox doctoring may serve as a catalyst to correct the problem, but it will not always correct the cause of the problem.

Modem medicine still is unsure of how various diseases manifest. Why do they affect some people and not others? What makes some people prone to illness and other imbalances? Words such as *virus*, *bacteria*, and *weakened constitution* are not really explanations. Viruses and bacteria surround us all the time, so why do we get sick sometimes and not others?

This book is not a manual to replace or substitute for orthodox medicine and doctoring. The methods are not, nor should they be taken as, prescriptive. They are simply descriptions of tried and true therapies used by others in the past. They have been used in conjunction with, in place of, and in varying combinations of orthodox medical treatments. All treatments, traditional or otherwise, have function and viability!

There are times when the orthodox medical approach (including surgery) is very necessary to the restoration of balance and health. To make it exclusive though, as a treatment, is to deny that a divine healing source operates within the universe. It is the same as saying that such a force is narrow-minded and prejudicial in its approach to humanity. It implies that healing can only come through certain individuals, for certain individuals.

If nothing else, this manual should provide an opportunity, for anyone willing to put forth the effort, to experience the innate healing ability that resides within us all without exception. It will demonstrate that we each can participate actively in the healing of our bodies by opening our perceptions, expanding our knowledge, and taking back the responsibility. We each can alleviate our pains and aches. We each can facilitate orthodox medical treatments and balance ourselves on all levels. We can heal our lives!

The techniques described in this book are guidelines only. They have been employed by many throughout history. They are learned abilities. You do not have to be "gifted" to use them. They are simple, practical, and do not require tremendous amounts of formal education. This is a manual for helping yourself. It is not a cure-all and be-all, but it will show you that you can control and heal more aspects of your life than you probably ever imagined.

There is a popular saying that "If you have your health, you have everything." Unfortunately, our health is something not appreciated until we are without it. Think about how many times you have promised yourself to change or improve a habit. Most of the time, these promises are made while ill or "down" with something. The moment we start to feel better, we forget it or let it slide. We ignore the fact that our body rebelled, thumped us on the head with an illness, to get our attention.

It takes effort to restore health and balance. Yes, the body has a natural ability to bounce back, but with time that ability can diminish, particularly if we do nothing to assist it. The human body can only do so much on its own. If we don't assist it, we may encounter health crises that demand more radical cures, and over time all we will be able to do is alleviate and not cure.

Working with vibrational healing traditions serves many functions. It opens our awareness of how we operate on more than just a physical level. It demonstrates tangibly that we can effect changes in body conditions through the proper use of holistic techniques. It shows us what we need to learn about ourselves, what we need to change about ourselves, and what we can control in ourselves.

The modern approach to medicine is in a vicious cycle. We develop a problem (in reality, a symptom of something larger) and we treat the symptom. It disappears, but later something else pops up. We treat it, and the cycle continues. There is no escape from this cycle as long as we continue to think of health in purely physical terms, and treat ill health by simply looking for a pill that will relieve us of the physical discomfort.

For true health, there is no "fast food" remedy. Yes, there are things that can be done to alleviate the discomfort of a runny nose, but it does not cure what made you susceptible to that runny nose. We must learn to realize that a runny nose is a means by which the body eliminates toxins from your system. It is part of the body's natural cleansing process. If we take a pill to stop the runny nose, we stop the body's cleansing. The toxins then accumulate until some later time when they trigger an even greater problem.

It is essential that we begin recognizing the forces and causes behind our illnesses. Learning about these and how they intimately play upon and affect our physical well-being is one of the major purposes for working with any of the healing arts. It involves more than just a spiritual faith that such techniques have merit. The techniques are based in physical reality, operating according to the natural laws of the universe.

Healing, as approached in this manual, includes the locating and removing of energy blockages wherever they occur—physical or otherwise. This requires a rise in consciousness and a greater understanding of the metaphysical nature of the human body and its energy system. Areas of the body in which energy is blocked (especially for extended periods) and misuse of our body creates dysfunction. This manual will show simple ways of restoring the natural flow of energy to the area that has been blocked or is dysfunctioning.

The ways and means of accomplishing this are many. Some require greater study and education, others not as much. The techniques in this book can be used by anyone—even those who know nothing of metaphysics—to experience the ability to heal, even if only to remove a headache. They are not complicated, magical, or beyond comprehension.

Once experienced, your life can never be the same. All the world takes on greater significance. Every thought, word, and deed takes on greater import as their interplay with the physical becomes concretely understood. You will begin to know that you control much of what you experience in the line of dis-ease and ill health. You will see the options open to you. You will become aware of life and energy operating on all planes and dimensions within you and around you.

Part of what we all must learn is that there is a divine spark within us. We are here to learn that life is supposed to go right. We are here to learn how to make it right. People receive answers to their prayers, experience a healing, and then exclaim, "The most amazing thing happened!" The truth is prayers are supposed to be answered. Miracles are supposed to happen. Healing is supposed to occur. The truly amazing thing would be if they did not!

When we were children, there were no limits. Everything was possible. We need to see the world sparkle again, as if for the first time. There is adventure and joy and magic yet to be born within our lives. It is the hope and wish of the author that through this work, you begin to experience a rebirth of the health and color and light within your own life, so that you can then become a light unto others!

part 1

HOLISTIC HEALTH AND THE HUMAN ESSENCE

A person will get well when he is tired of being sick.

Lao Tzu in the *Tao te Ching*

one

HOLISTIC HEALTH

Health is the ideal balance between all major parts of our being (body, mind, and soul) in conjunction with our environment and all we encounter. The word *healing* has its roots in the Greek *holos* from which we get *whole* or *holistic*. Healing is wholeness, but not just wholeness as expressed and experienced in physical life. It encompasses our whole essence: physical, emotional, mental, and spiritual. To ignore any one aspect is to deprive yourself of health.

All paths of spiritual development tell us to look within. For all matters of health, we must do likewise. All healing comes from within! The body heals itself. This healing can be initiated from an outside source, though, that serves to set the healing process in motion.

Before any true healing can occur, there are certain prerequisites:

The individual must understand his/her own basic health patterns—including strengths and weaknesses.
We must come to know our body and its response to outside influences, its basic strengths and weaknesses, what we can handle and what we cannot. A dis-ease manifestation most often occurs in a weak area of the body. This weakened area can be the result of stress or even a susceptibility due to the basic genetics of the individual.

3

This susceptibility is not the same as being "destined to be sick." We have free will, and even though we may have a biologically weak area within our body's make-up, it does not mean that dis-ease and illness will manifest. If we are aware of such weaknesses and susceptibilities, we can take measures to strengthen them and protect ourselves from imbalance. Despite the role of genetics in forming basic health patterns, we still have a tremendous ability to effect changes in those patterns. We must come to understand how all aspects of our body operate.

The individual must learn to see all physical conditions as symptoms.

All physical imbalance, dis-ease, and illness are symptoms only. There is something else—be it an emotional or mental pattern, stress, etc.— that has promoted and instigated the physical symptom.

Often we ignore our negative patterns and imbalances until we are thumped on the head with them. In most cases, the physical dis-ease is a hearty "call to attention" by the physical body. It is the body's way of telling us that something has gotten out of balance.

The individual must take responsibility and seek out alternatives that affect the whole being.

We must be willing to widen our perspectives and implement the alternatives necessary to restore health and balance on all levels. Such alternatives are not always quick and easy, but if implemented correctly, they are often effective in eliminating the symptoms and their causes.

There are always alternatives. There are many methods of healing, many therapies, and many remedies. We each must find the method or combination of methods that suit our own energy system, physical and otherwise. Sometimes we must borrow from several modalities to come up with a synthesis that is uniquely effective for us. The important factor is finding the combination of methods that is most beneficial at the time we need it.

In discovering the alternatives that work for you, you must consider all aspects of your being. Your emotions, your thought patterns, and your spiritual perspectives are as important to your health as the physical state of the various systems, tissues, and organs of the body. Whether you are concerned about being healthy, regaining health, or moving to greater health and energy, the whole being—physical and subtle—must be involved.

The individual must employ common sense in the maintenance of balanced health.

Many that venture out upon spiritual paths have a tendency to ignore the physical. There exists the misconception that if you are living a spiritual life, it will automatically take care of the physical. The truth is both must go hand in hand. All the ancient scriptures speak of the body being a temple. That temple needs care. No matter how spiritual your thoughts are, if you do not give proper care to the physical temple, problems will arise. This proper care should at the very least include:

a. Proper diet

b. Proper exercise

c. Proper rest

d. Proper breathing

You can be the most gifted and spiritual person alive, but if you do not employ all four of these in your care of the body, disease will manifest.

Metaphysical Awareness of Health

We are multidimensional beings. We operate from physical, emotional, mental, and spiritual dimensions simultaneously. For true health to occur, we must begin to learn how these dimensions all interact and affect our overall health patterns.

Metaphysical means beyond the physical. It implies a causation beyond the physical. As humans we have a tendency to look at ourselves from a limited perspective. We are encased in flesh. We may speak of the soul or the spirit, but we are physical creatures. We think, feel, act, and react from a physical awareness, but we are more than just physical beings. Those thoughts and feelings, although not tangibly physical, do affect physical conditions and perspectives. They are a dimension to our essence that very strongly affects our physical well-being.

Most dis-ease stems from a metaphysical base. It does not usually originate in the physical body or in the environment. Those things of the physical environment that we attribute to dis-ease most often (viruses, bacteria, etc.) are around us all the time. It is our metaphysical aspects, though, that make us susceptible to their manifesting a problem. Imbalanced emotions, attitudes, and thoughts will deplete our natural physical energies and immunities so that we are more likely to "catch a cold" or manifest some other problem. Even when illness results from lack of exercise or poor diet, the emotional and mental causes of such habits should be explored.

In the ancient Hebrew mysticism know as the Qabala, specific names were given for how God manifests and works within the universe and through humanity. Operating at the heart of the universe—at the heart of the Tree of Life—is the divine name Jehovah Aloah ve-Daath. This name can be freely translated as "God made manifest in the sphere of the mind." At the heart of our lives, at the heart of our health and well-being, is the mind. What we think sets the energy in motion for what we will experience, particularly in regard to our health.

Inside each of us is a level of our subconscious that responds literally, like a child, to all of our thoughts and expressions. This level also works to maintain our health. It takes our thoughts, feelings, and expressions, and sets them in motion so they can manifest. When we make such statements as "I get two colds every winter," that aspect of the mind begins working with our physical energy. Then, as winter approaches, we are more susceptible to catch those two colds. Our thoughts, feelings, and words become self-fulfilling prophecies, often playing themselves out within the physical body itself.

That level of the subconscious directs much of what manifests in our bodies and our environments. It responds literally to our thoughts, feelings, and expressions. You tell friends that you "lost ten pounds" and that inner child, that level of the subconscious, perks up its ears. "Lost? Lost?" The subconscious immediately begins working to find those ten pounds you lost, and it usually throws in a few extra, just in case you lose them again.

If we are constantly yelling and criticizing that inner child, it's no wonder our lives do not work. None of us want to be around some-one who is always criticizing us. Do we want to yell at that child within, or do we want to nurture and love it? This is what responsi-bility in healing is about.

Our health is our choice. Some may say they can't help how they feel and think about themselves. They complain that it's what they have experienced their whole life. And that is sad, but it's sadder still if we choose to continue those patterns when we can change them. We can't change the past, but our future—particularly our future health—is being shaped by our current thoughts and feelings. If we change our imaginings, we change our world.

As we begin to work with healing energies, it will become increas-ingly apparent that most imbalances arise from some expression of nonlove toward ourselves. It is easy to recognize those expressions if we look for them. We scold and criticize ourselves. We tell ourselves that we are too fat, too thin, too old, too young, too short, too tall. We drink or take drugs. We refuse to exercise. We eat wrong. We blame ourselves for everything. We compare ourselves to others. We fail to make decisions. We constantly rehash past mistakes. We assume we're not good enough to do the things we would like to do.

We must begin to realize that only we are responsible for our thoughts and feelings, only we will suffer their consequences, good, bad, or indifferent. If we continue to focus upon the negative, we create imbalance within our emotional and mental beings, and these will work themselves into an imbalance within our physical body as well.

While most orthodox doctors deal primarily with the physical, a healer will deal with all aspects of a person's energy. A true healer will work to correct the physical symptom and its underlying, metaphysical cause.

A healer is one who learns to attune to vital, curative forces—physical and spiritual—so as to be a conductor of healing energy. The ability to conduct such healing energy is a learned ability, and it can be developed by anyone wishing to enhance his/her own well-being. The degree to which it is conducted determines the degree of healing that occurs. (See the chart on natural and spiritual healing agencies on the facing page.)

Inherent within this is the understanding that for the healing to occur, the individual receiving the healing energies must desire to be healed. Unfortunately, many people enjoy being sick. They enjoy the attention. They enjoy having an excuse for doing or not doing certain things in their lives. They enjoy having something to blame their own sense of failure on: "If I hadn't been so sick, I could have accomplished so much."

For many, being sick is a way of giving up without having to publicly admit it or face the assumed failures. Society accepts illness as a legitimate excuse. This is why I have heard cancer called the acceptable form of suicide. We can manifest this, and not have the stigma of suicide attached to it. In fact, individuals can leave the world while giving the impression that they are fighters and noble in the face of death. For some, it is nothing more than a way of relieving oneself of the responsibility of life.

On the other hand, the illness may manifest for other reasons, and we must be careful about jumping to conclusions or pointing fingers in accusation. Everyone's case is unique, and one person's form of suffering is no more significant than someone else's. The important factor is in discovering the cause or causes of what is creating the physical imbalance.

Sample Natural and Spiritual Curative Agencies

The Natural Agencies	*The Spiritual Agencies*
Medicines	Prayer
Massage	Meditation
Manipulation (e.g., Rolfing)	Creative visualization
Corrective physical exercise	Self-realization
Psychotherapeutics	Healing angels/guides
Chiropractic methods	Invocations
Herbal remedies	Spiritual blessings
Surgery	Dreamwork
Acupuncture and acupressure	Past-life therapy
Homeopathy	Faith
Diet	Affirmations
Radionics	Others
Trager	
Reiki	
Polarity therapy	
Rebirthing	
Exercise (yoga, tai chi, etc.)	
Etheric/therapeutic touch	
Aromatherapy	
Color and light therapy	
Sound	
Vitamin therapy	
Flower essences	
Others	

People put themselves in the position to manifest an illness, creating sickness for many reasons:

- To force themselves to grow and learn.

- To foster compassion in themselves and others.

- To learn something about personal responsibility.

- To provide a means for that transition we call death.

- To get love and attention from others.

- To help teach others.

- To stimulate a new perception of life and its processes.

- To cleanse the body of toxins accumulated from sources outside of itself (i.e., pollutants, etc.).

Each person's reason(s) is unique to themselves, and part of the healer's responsibility is to help uncover the patterns that triggered the physical imbalance.

The physical body has a natural ability to maintain a steady, balanced, internal state within certain limits or parameters. This is called *homeostasis*.

We incarnate under various conditions to test this homeostasis, and to develop a greater ability at maintaining it. It is why we encounter so much trial and error and change within our lives. By learning to flow with the rhythms of our life and still maintain balance, our energies grow. When we hold ourselves back from experiencing life and its changes—for good or bad—we create stress that will internalize. This internalized stress is the primary cause of all sickness.

Every dis-ease has a positive aspect to it. The ailment provides an indicator as to where we are out of balance or where there is stress in our life. It helps us to recognize the negative energies we are cultivating on other levels of our being. Through the holistic healing process, we learn the cause and its inherent lessons, bringing the body back into balance. If we fail to get to the cause, we only alleviate symptoms.

In such cases these imbalanced energies within the body will look for another outlet. The illness will remanifest, either in another way or another place, and usually more intensely.

Modern pharmaceuticals are directed against symptoms. They act swiftly and powerfully to remove the symptoms and the signs of the real dis-ease in the body. They do bring superficial relief, but it is little more than a "fast food" remedy. They alleviate the inconvenience of the illness temporarily. They relieve the individual from having to take the time and responsibility of correcting the cause.

This can create problems down the road, as it pushes aside the warning signals that we are internalizing some stress. This is most evident in the way we treat colds within Western society. That runny nose is inconvenient and bothersome, but it is also the way the body cleans toxins from its system. If we take medications to stop the runny nose, we stop the body from cleansing itself. We are preventing the toxins from being removed from the body.

The body occasionally goes through what is called a *healing crisis*. This often occurs just when an individual is working to consciously reshape his/her health. We may begin a regimen of exercise, good eating habits, etc., and then after a few weeks we find ourselves down with the flu or some other similar illness. This is the beginning of the healing crisis, a process for cleansing the body and strengthening it. The body is responding to your efforts to improve its health.

The things we are exposed to, along with our own bad habits, create toxins in the body. These toxins settle into the body like a sludge at the bottom of the river. As we work to bring our body into health, that sludge gets stirred up. It gets brought to the surface, but this is so we can sift it off and leave ourselves more vibrant and energetic. Unfortunately, many people use this as an excuse to cease their efforts. We need to see this as a signal that our efforts are being rewarded and that the body is responding. Yes, it is troublesome initially, but if allowed to run its course it will leave us stronger.

Healing crises occur whenever the body needs to be cleansed. The body will choose a time when it knows it will have enough vitality to stand the shock. Healing crises often occur when a person is feeling best, and when he/she has time to spare. (It's amazing how many people get sick during vacations.) If we maintain conscious efforts to improve, the body will remove toxins and waste from the system in a natural manner, without the disruption of a healing crisis.

There is also what is sometimes termed a *dis-ease crisis*. This occurs when the body is full of toxins, waste, and mucus. It is clogged to the limit. This crisis can occur in many ways. We may have ignored all prior warning signals, and there are always warning signals! We may have abused our bodies with lack of sleep, improper diet, little or no exercise, etc. When the body becomes clogged enough, the germs begin to multiply. The toxicity of the body intensifies and seeks out its weakest area(s).

Illness occurs when the body strength and vitality is lowest. The dis-ease crisis kicks in as a means to save your life. It is a forced cleansing, a very powerful cleansing because there is manifesting injury to body organs, cancerous conditions, poisons in the blood, or some other traumatic condition. Such an illness can last several weeks or even months. Much of it depends upon how long we have ignored the proper maintenance.

It is not unusual to find dis-ease crises being triggered when the weather gets colder. When the physical body becomes cold, everything contracts. In essence, this forces an elimination of the toxins. Such a crisis usually lays the individual up to where self-assessment and self-evaluation begins to occur. This is why heart attacks and manifestations of cancer, for example, will cause a dramatic change in lifestyle. The crisis forces a reckoning and reevaluation.

The ancient healers recognized the importance of treating the whole person, not just symptoms. They recognized the importance of paying attention to everything. They recognized the importance of knowing how the body functions, and thus they were able to use methods that promoted its natural functions. They recognized the importance of the spiritual growth of the individual in the healing process. Dis-ease on any level gives us an opportunity to learn and thus reach a higher state of awareness and consciousness. The process we use in our own healing reflects our ability to move into new perspectives.

The Zen Buddhists have a wonderful three-line poem that reflects this:

> I chop wood. I carry water.
> This is my magic.

Inherent within this poem is the recognition that everything in the physical is a miracle. It is magic because our essence is a spiritual essence that is manifesting through a physical body. And if we can manifest something as magnificent as the human body, we can certainly manifest a little better health, abundance, prosperity, and fulfillment within our lives.

An old occult axiom states "All energy follows thought." Where we place our thoughts, that is where energy will begin to manifest. If we change our imaginings, we change our world. We must begin to dwell upon the infinite possibilities, rewards, blessings, and potentials that are possible within our lives, rather than how limited we are. As we learn to do so, we find that we do not have to be at the mercy of our life circumstances or our bodies. We can bring light, energy, and health into our lives and into the lives of all we touch. And that is becoming a healer.

two

THE OCCULT SIGNIFICANCE
OF THE BODY

Our body is more than a simple physical shell comprised of organs et al. It has a significance much greater than we often imagine. All energies upon the earth and those of the heavens play themselves out through it. Seeing the body as more than just a physical instrument that enables us to exist is crucial to empowering ourselves and enhancing our health.

Our body is a microcosm. It is a universe of energies unto itself. It reflects the greater energies of the universe—the macrocosm. When humans are called a microcosm, it should not infer that we are just a part of the universe, but rather that we are a miniature universe.

This means our hands are not just instruments for grabbing and holding on. Our legs are not just for standing and moving. Our heart is not just for pumping blood. Every part of our body has a significance much greater than its physical responsibilities.

Every aspect of our body has an occult or hidden significance. These are points that the energies of the universe flow through and manifest. They are points in which our own mental, emotional, and spiritual attitudes and energies have dynamic play.

Heavenly Associations with the Body

Planet/Sign	Parts of Body Ruled
Sun	heart, back
Moon	stomach, breasts, digestion
Mercury	hands, arms, nervous system, solar plexus
Venus	throat, voice, loins, veins, kidneys
Mars	head, sex organs, muscular system
Jupiter	hips, thighs, liver
Saturn	skeletal system, knees, teeth
Uranus	ankles, shins, cerebro-spinal system
Neptune	feet
Pluto	generative organs
Aries	head, face
Taurus	neck, throat
Gemini	hands, lungs
Cancer	breasts, stomach
Leo	heart
Virgo	intestines
Libra	kidneys, ovaries
Scorpio	sex organs
Sagittarius	hips, thighs
Capricorn	knees
Aquarius	ankles, calves
Pisces	feet

We are susceptible to influence from all energies around us. This includes the energies from that which we ingest in some form (food, air, drink, etc.), as well as those energies outside of us to which we are exposed (people, environments, attitudes, sounds, etc.).

Our body is an energy resonator and monitor. It has the capacity to resonate with almost any form of energy, positive or negative.

Under normal conditions, the body has a natural ability to throw off negative influences before problems can develop.

The body also monitors the energies we are exposed to by providing us with physical feedback through symptoms. If we are exposed to positive influences and energies, we become stronger and more energized. If we are overly exposed to negative influences, we lose energy, develop aches or illnesses, or manifest some dis-ease in a physical form. Our body informs us of a problem area within our body and also in our life. Where the problem manifests provides the clues as to the source of the problem.

Begin by examining and learning what the various body parts and systems do. Learn their physical functions. Then examine any occult significance that could be applied to them. Ask yourself, "What could this symbolize or signify?" For example, if we are having difficulty with cramps in our hands, we find that cramps involve an unrelaxed contraction of a muscle. In regard to the hands then, is there something or someone we may be trying to cling to, or hold onto too tightly? Do we need to relax our grip on some idea, person, or goal? Whatever it is, it is not beneficial for us, or we would not be experiencing the negative symptom of the cramps.

When we work to determine the cause of a problem or disease and what it can teach us, we need to examine three aspects:

- We need to examine the physical symptom that is manifesting and its hidden significance.

- We must look at the organ or body part in which the symptom is revealing itself. This includes examining its normal healthy function as well as its dysfunction.

- We should also examine the system that the organ or body part belongs to, including its hidden significance as well.

The more we know about all three, the easier it will be to eliminate the physical symptom and its root cause so that it cannot create future problems for us as well. We will be able to heal ourselves and enlighten ourselves simultaneously. Remember that we can learn something from every dis-ease.

The Occult Significance of Specific Symptoms

The symptoms we experience in our dis-ease can tell us much of the emotional, mental, and spiritual states that have helped the imbalance to manifest. The following are not diagnostic. They are descriptions of common symptoms experienced for various health imbalances. The hidden significances associated with them are not all-inclusive. They are simply designed to give you a starting point in examining those elements in your life, which help to create dis-ease. They should help trigger specific insights into your own unique condition.

Keep in mind that most symptoms have physical causes that must be rooted out. For example, cramps can be caused by a lack of calcium in the diet. We can help correct the problem by including more calcium, but if we do not get to what made us ignore our calcium intake, the problem is more likely to resurface again somewhere down the road.

Yes, the physical symptom must be dealt with from a physical level, but there is also a metaphysical cause that assisted that problem in manifesting. We must try and determine what emotional, mental, or spiritual conditions have assisted in allowing the physical dis-ease to manifest. If we don't, we are practicing a band-aid type of health care instead of taking a holistic, preventive approach.

Chills and Fevers

Chills are sensations of coldness, usually accompanied by shivering. They often occur at intervals with fevers. A fever is an abnormal or undue rise in body temperature, often accompanied by a quickening of the pulse. These two symptoms reflect the body working to shake off, burn off, and realign itself.

Two basic precepts of physics are reflected in symptoms of chills and fevers. If we wish to convert matter into spirit, we must raise its energy or apply heat. If we wish to convert spirit into matter, we must condense it, such as drawing it down through the application of coldness. For example, to turn ice into steam, we apply heat. To convert steam into ice, we apply cold.

A fever reflects the conversion of matter to spirit. The raising of the temperature and the quickening of the pulse are designed to heat up and burn off the toxins in the physical body. This conversion of toxins through fever is a form of elimination. It also allows our subtle bodies to extend away from the physical body to draw more energy into and through them to enhance the healing process. (See the references to the subtle bodies in the following chapter.)

A chill reflects the conversion of spirit to matter, or an aligning of spirit and matter more fully. The shivering that often accompanies chills is a means of drawing the subtle bodies back into alignment with the physical.

If we experience stronger symptoms of fevers, it can tell us that we are losing touch with the spiritual. It can reflect a toxic congestion with physical matters. It can indicate the need to stimulate the physical body into greater activity, to raise the pulse. Have you been more sedentary lately? Have you not been acting upon things as you should? Have you been allowing things to sit and accumulate? Have you neglected aspects of yourself other than the physical? Are things heating up around you and you are not acting upon them? Are your desires heating up and not being expressed? Are you holding in anger about something, so that it has to try and release itself from the physical before a problem arises?

If we are experiencing chills, it can reflect a number of possibilities as well. Chills cause contraction, a pulling in. Are you in some way pulling into yourself? Are you pulling in, away from something? Have you been more scattered and flaky lately, needing to pull in and ground yourself? Have you been involved in so many activities that you have left no time for yourself? Are things and activities about you scattered and disorganized? Are you trying to shake some new order into your life? Is there so much activity that you are having difficulty absorbing it all? Have you been feeling insecure, "left out in the cold" in some area of your life?

Congestion

Congestion is a condition in which an area of the body becomes filled to excess or overburdened. It is an excessive accumulation of blood, mucus, etc., in the vessels of an organ or a part of an organ. Sinuses and lungs are the most common places of congestion, although constipation is also a form of congestion.

Where the congestion occurs can tell us much about what we are overburdening ourselves with. If our head is congested, what does this tell us of our thought processes? Are we allowing irritation to build within us? Are our worries, doubts, and fears filling our head, congesting it?

If the congestion occurs in the lungs, creating breathing problems, this can tell us much as well. Are we holding in our emotions? Lung congestion can reflect a suppressed or inner crying that needs to be brought out. Are we refusing to allow more things and people in our life or is this being prevented by others? Are we not feeling the right to take up space and so are congesting ourselves? Is there depression or sadness that is filling the heart and not being expressed? This also can cause congestion. Are we afraid to take in life (breath), and so congest the lungs to prevent ourselves from doing so? Are we feeling stifled or doing some stifling in some way?

Constipation is also a form of congestion. It often reflects a refusal to eliminate old ideas, emotions, and patterns that are no longer beneficial. Individuals that are stuck in the past and refuse to change often experience varying degrees of constipation.

Cramps

Cramps are sudden, involuntary contractions of a muscle or group of muscles. Many physical conditions can cause cramps, ranging from a lack of calcium in the system, to exercising a muscle vigorously without a warm-up, to a lack of food or oxygen.

There are also metaphysical conditions that can help put us in a position to manifest cramps. With cramps, there is a strong contraction of the muscle. It is a drawing in, a holding on. This is often a response of fear or a refusal to take time to relax. It reflects tension, a holding in of everything.

Where the cramps occur can tell you much. Cramps in the hands may tell you that you are trying to hold on too tightly to something or that you don't want to let yourself go. Your body, through the cramping, is telling you that you need to relax and let go. If in the legs, it may be telling you that you are moving and working too much. It is not unusual to find individuals who are workaholics and "supermoms" experiencing cramps in the hands and legs.

Menstrual cramps are not quite as easy to pinpoint. With many women, the intensity of the cramps varies from month to month. An examination of activities, emotions, and general life experiences over several months will help pinpoint problem areas. Menstrual cramps can reflect issues centered around one's own femininity and should be reflected upon as well.

Fatigue

Fatigue is very simply telling us that we are tired, but not just on a physical level. It can reflect a "tired of life" attitude that has begun to affect the physical energy levels. What are you really tired of in your life: your job, your partner, the constant stress from the family, etc.?

When there is a lack of love for your activities, fatigue creeps in. Are you not taking time to include enjoyable, fun activities in your life? Have you forgotten that the human essence needs playtime? Sometimes fatigue will arise to encourage us to find ways of playing.

Infection

Infections are a sign that poisons or toxins are in the body or a part of the body. Infections can reflect or reveal negativity, anger, and fears that are beginning to affect the physical life of the individual, making us more susceptible to infection or its spread. Are there "toxic" thoughts,

fears, and worries that you are harboring and nursing? Is there disharmony and negativity around you that you are allowing to affect you?
Are you permitting yourself to be exposed to negative and unhealthy
people, situations, environs? What bad habits are we fostering that may
be allowing toxins to accumulate?

To infect means "to affect or contaminate (a person, organ, wound,
etc.) with disease-producing germs" and "to taint or contaminate with
something that affects the quality, character, or condition unfavorably."[1] This definition should tell us how to approach the examination
of any infection we have manifested. Who or what has been affecting
the quality, character, and condition of your life unfavorably recently?

Inflammation

Inflammation reveals itself in the human body through "redness,
swelling, pain, tenderness, heat, and a generally disturbed function
of an area of the body, usually as a reaction to an injurious agent."[2]
This definition provides many clues to the occult significance of any
inflammation that occurs in our life.

What injurious agent (person, condition, attitude, negativity, etc.)
have you been exposing yourself to? Have you been harboring an-
noyance and aggravation at individuals and situations? Is there anger
and frustration that you have not found a proper outlet for? What is
intruding upon and preventing feelings of peacefulness and calm
within your life? Are you angry and frustrated with your life or some
specific life conditions? Are you being overly critical of yourself or
exposing yourself to those who are overly critical of you? Do you not
approve of yourself at this time for some reason? Are you refusing to
change old patterns (especially if the inflammation recurs)?

---

1 Stein, Jess, editor-in-chief. *Random House Dictionary of the English Language*
  (New York: Random House), 1970.

2 Ibid.

Irritation

Irritations are a lesser degree of inflammation in many ways. Some of the symptoms are the same, but irritations also could include burning and itching. The same questions for inflammations should also be asked for irritations.

Is something "burning you up" and aggravating you in your life? Is there an unexpressed desire or unfulfilled wish (an itch) that you are not acting upon? Are you literally itching to do something but not acting upon it? Where is there dissatisfaction in your life? What is unresolved and so still burns or itches? Who or what is most irritating to you at the time? Is there a fear that your needs and desires will be unfulfilled? Are you not happy with your present position in life?

Nausea

Nausea is a sickness or queasiness of the stomach. It can be accompanied by the involuntary impulse to vomit. There is much hidden significance in this, and examining our own life when we experience this symptom can reveal tremendous insight.

What are we sick of in our life? What attitude(s) have we been exposed to that we do not want to digest? What are we trying to throw off or expel (in the case of vomiting)? Is there a fear of rejection? Is there a rejection to someone or something? Are we not feeling safe and secure? Are we having difficulty swallowing something?

Pain

Pain comes in many forms and disguises, and so it can be difficult at times to pinpoint those areas that have aggravated and helped manifest the pain we are experiencing. In general, it can reflect such feelings as guilt, nursing old hurts, overly critical attitudes by others or ourselves, longings, resistance to new moves and changes, and feelings of a lack of freedom.

The location of the pain can provide much insight. Is it a headache? If so, maybe it has to do with what we are thinking about ourselves. If it is a heartache, maybe it reflects our feelings or lack of feelings for ourselves and even a lack of expression of love. It is not unusual for someone who talks of another being a "pain in the neck" to develop soreness and stiffness of the neck.

Pain can be chronic or acute. Chronic pain often recurs and persists. With chronic pain and conditions, we often find a refusal to change. It can reflect longstanding fears and overworn patterns of behavior. An acute pain is sharp, and often severe and intense. It reflects a drastic call to attention by the body. Both can reflect sensitivity to criticism and being overwhelmed by details.

Examine your pain. Is it achy? Throbbing? Steady? Sharp? All can provide clues as to what may be lying behind the physical symptom itself. Are you longing for something? Do you long for love? Are you not approving of yourself or do not feel the approval of others? Are you punishing yourself or feeling guilty? Are you being overly critical, not being gentle enough with yourself? Are you restricting yourself or your activities unnecessarily? Who or what is really being a pain in your life at this time? If it is chronic, who or what is always a pain in your life?

Swelling

Swelling often indicates a clogged attitude or process in life. Those who are stuck in old patterns often find they have repeated problems with swelling. The body area affected can reflect much. For example, swollen ankles, such as through water retention, can reflect a refusal to move on (the water is not circulating), or it can reflect a refusal to let others move on.

Swelling can also reflect being stuck in outworn patterns and ideas. It can also reflect issues surrounding self-esteem. Are we being too puffed up about something? Are we not expanding and growing when we have the opportunities (and thus, the swelling and growth becomes clogged internally)? Are we inflating things out of proportion? Are we becoming too emotional and not allowing common sense and practical thinking to be utilized? Are we protruding into others' lives or areas where we should not be?

These are just some of the symptoms and some of their significances. Examination of your own will elicit specific insights. Don't become superstitious in this process of analysis. For example, if a happy, healthy child cuts his/her foot while playing and develops a slight infection, don't assume that the child helped manifest this problem. Accidents do happen and not everything can be controlled while we are in the physical, but much of it can. The more we become aware of it, the healthier we will stay. We should try to learn something about ourselves and how our physical body responds to what we are exposed to in the world every time a dis-ease manifests.

Some Occult Significances of the Body

Not only do symptoms reflect other forces or energies at work in our life, but the body part or organ that experiences the symptom can provide even further insight. The body has often been viewed as a microcosm, as a unique symbol for the expression of certain forces within our life. The body part or organ can reflect where those forces or energies are being expressed or experienced in an unbalanced manner.

Study the parts of the body. Become familiar with their functions and the systems they belong to. This can provide clues as to how balanced or unbalanced we work with natural propensities.

The following descriptions are not all-inclusive. They are simply a guideline for you to begin your own self-examination. They will help you in beginning to take back upon yourself the responsibility for your own health and life.

Ankles

This is the joint connecting the feet and the legs. It is a point at which movement can occur forward and/or upward. The ankles are the symbol for support in your movements. Are they strong or weak? What does this say about your own movements or lack of movement in life?

The right angle they form between the feet and the lower part of the legs is significant. It reflects operating in two dimensions or two planes. They are symbols to remind us to move forward on the physical while reaching for the spiritual. Are we working in both levels? Are we trying to lead a cloistered existence? Are we staying grounded while we work on our spiritual evolvement? Are we ignoring the spiritual and becoming too immersed in the physical? Are we not wanting or resisting movement in a specific direction in our life?

Anus

This is the opening for excretion to occur. It is the point in the body where we let go of waste and that which is no longer usable by the body. It is the symbol of release and letting go. Pain in this area can reflect an aching to release something or someone, as can itching.

Are we holding onto that which is no longer beneficial? Are we trying to hold onto the past? Are we letting life rush by us, watching but not participating fully? Are we feeling overburdened or afraid to let go? Are we rejecting what life is offering us? Are we feeling rejected by someone or something in our life?

Arms

This upper limb of the body is a symbol of our ability to embrace and hold life experiences. It is a symbol of activity, work, and play. Strong arms reflect an ability to handle activities well, along with an ability to reach for new heights.

If we have problems with our arms, is it because we are overextending our reach? Are we not extending it out when we should? Are we wanting to strike out? Are we blaming others for that which we can't reach or hold onto? Are we trying to shoulder too much responsibility? Are we giving away our responsibility? Are we feeling things are hopeless and we are beyond help? Do we feel as if we won't be able to pull ourselves through certain situations?

Bladder (Gall)

The gall bladder is a small sac in which bile secreted by the liver is stored until needed for the process of fat digestion. Problems in this area can indicate we are trying to digest things too quickly or are not digesting what we have experienced; we are not learning our lessons. Such problems as gallstones can indicate we are holding onto hard thoughts and bitter experiences rather than moving past them. We are holding onto the past and allowing it to fill our life, rather than moving forward with joy and anticipation to the future.

Bladder (Urinary)

The urinary bladder is a smooth muscle sac that is integral to the elimination of urine from the body. Problems in this area usually are amplified and manifested through anxiety and anger. Are you "pissed off" at someone? Is someone "pissed off" at you? Weak bladders often stem from fears, often childhood fears that are never fully resolved. Fear of letting go of the past or what is no longer beneficial (even if it is familiar, and thus safe) can cause bladder problems. An attitude of "better the devil you know than the one you don't" can cause elimination problems, especially affecting the urinary bladder.

Blood

This is the life fluid of the individual. It has great importance and great hidden significance as well. It represents the flow of life energy. It contains the life essence and pattern of the individual, past and present, which is partly why it was often a part of ancient mystical rites. It represents the vitality and joy of life.

Such conditions as high and low blood pressure have hidden significance as well. High blood pressure often reflects longstanding and unresolved emotional problems or turmoil. The past is not being released; it is simply and continually kept at a low boil. It is not unusual to find individuals with high blood pressure stuck in old, worn-out patterns and emotions and not moving on. Low blood pressure can reflect fear and/or apathy to movement in life. A "what's the use" attitude is common. Blood infections and anemia are common as well.

Blood infections should be examined as well. What toxic thoughts are we allowing to infect our vitality? Are we dissipating our primal vital forces in an unhealthy manner (bad or negative habits)? With anemia, there is a deficiency of red blood cells. In such cases, are we limiting vital activities in our life? Are we afraid to let go and enjoy life?

Bones

Bones are the support system of the body. They are the foundation and structure. They have been symbols for the seeds of life and even of resurrection. Problems with bones tell us that there is something wrong in an area of our life's foundation and structure. We may need to rebuild, rebalance, restrengthen, or completely restructure. It can also indicate problems with authority.

The spine is often likened to the great Tree of Life. It is the main support of the body. Are we not receiving the support we need from others? Are we not giving the support others need from us? What kind of support are we lacking or needing: financial, loving, emotional, sexual, etc.? Do we feel like others are "always on our back"? Are we trying to carry too much on our own backs? Are we not living the courage of our convictions, demonstrating "no spine"?

Brain

The brain is the main computer in our nervous system. It is the center of thought, memory, analysis, intuition, etc. Thus, the area of the brain affected can provide clues as to where we may be creating problems. There were many ancient beliefs that the brain and the skull were the doorways by which the spirit leaves at death and enters at birth. Physical problems can reflect problems in our thought processes. Are we holding onto thoughts that are not beneficial? Are our thoughts malignant? Are our thoughts distorted?

Breasts

The breasts are the milk-secreting organs of the body in the female. They are symbols of nurturing, nourishment, mothering, and sexuality. If we are having problems in this area of the body, we need to ask ourselves questions as to what made us more susceptible to them. Have we been "nursing old wounds"? Are we grieving or forgetting to grieve (remember the tradition of beating one's breast in mourning)? Are we feeling undernurtured by those we love? Are we afraid of growing up and maturing (as reflected in breast development)? Are we overmothering or smothering those around us? Are we not allowing ourselves to develop in the manner best for us?

Ears

The ears are the organs by which we hear. They also serve as centers for maintaining balance. If problems arise, what is it we do not want to hear? What is it we wish to hear but do not? Is there too much activity so that we cannot truly discern what is going on? Are we not listening to that inner voice when we should? Do we allow the words and actions of others to disrupt or disturb our own balance? Do we follow the words of others rather than our own inner voice? Are we trying to isolate ourselves or are we feeling isolated by others? Are we being too stubborn, refusing to hear any side but our own, or are we constantly around others like that?

Eyes

The eyes are our means for seeing. They are the symbols of vision and clairvoyance. They are the windows to the soul. If our vision is blurred, what are we not wishing to see? What do we have a distorted perception about? If our vision clouds (such as with cataracts), what are we clouding out of our life? Do we see no sunshine in our present or our future?

If we are farsighted, do we have difficulty looking at those things closest to us? Are we too focused on the future, the unmanifest? As many get older, the lens in the eye becomes more rigid, creating farsightedness. As we get older are we becoming more rigid, less flexible in our lives?

In nearsightedness, we see things clearly that are near but not those that are far. Are we becoming too focused on our self? Are we refusing to see the "big picture"? Are we afraid to look ahead to the future?

Feet

The feet are our support system. They enable us to stand and to move with ease. They are at the ground level of the body, at the foundation of our structure. The feet are symbols of stability and firmness. They help us to move upright. If we are having problems, what is changing around us in life? Is our foundation slipping? Are we refusing to move when we have the opportunity? Are we moving into areas we shouldn't? Is our basic understanding of ourselves and our lives weak? Are we not being as upright as we should? Are there others around us who are walking all over us, stepping on our feet? Do we need to take a firmer stand in our life?

Hands and Fingers

These are our tools for touching, caressing, and handling life's experiences. We use them to give and take, to attract and repel, to grasp or to push away. They can be raised in benediction or in anger. In traditional symbolism, the position of the hand was what was significant, and each finger had its own meaning.

If problems arise, are we refusing to touch or be touched by others? Are we holding too tightly onto something or someone? Are we releasing when we shouldn't be? Are we feeling victimized in some way? Are we allowing others to handle us and love affairs when we should be doing it ourselves? Are we intruding and handling the affairs of others when we shouldn't?

Heart

The heart is the primary organ of the circulatory system. It is the seat of life and the soul. It is the center for healing and loving. It is the sun center of the body. It is an ancient symbol for our feelings and emotions. It contains and works with our lifeblood.

Heart problems often reflect problems with the way in which we handle, experience, and/or express love and emotions. Are we hardened toward someone or something? Are we constricting our love or feeling it constricted by others? Are we limiting the joy in our life? Are we allowing our emotions and love to be the brunt of attack by others? Do we attack the manner in which others love, openly or internally? Do we feel we have to always give love and show love, even to those who don't appreciate it or acknowledge it? Do we believe we must always be working and struggling and sacrificing ourselves for others? Do we have an unhealthy concept of martyrdom in our life?

Hips and Buttocks

The hips and buttocks are symbols of balance, sexuality, and power. The hips particularly are important to the balance of the body, especially in forward movement. Problems with the hips may reflect problems in moving forward in our life. Are we unbalanced or unsure of our next movements? Are we allowing fear to restrict our movement forward?

The hips and buttocks are strong symbols of power and sexuality. If they are firm, it can reflect a firm and balanced sense of one's own power and sexuality in life. Loose and fleshy hips and buttocks may reflect insecurity in regard to one's power and sexuality. Are we hesitant to move forward? Are we not moving forward as strongly as we could? Are we expending our energies and power in unproductive endeavors?

Intestines

The intestines are part of the digestive system of the body. They are the lower part of the alimentary canal. The small intestines work to digest and absorb nutrients and the large intestines absorb water and eliminate the residue of digestion.

Problems in the intestinal tract often reflect problems in absorbing and eliminating elements and experiences in our life. Are we not learning what we need to be learning? Are lessons repeating themselves? Just as with indigestion, food will repeat on us. Do we hang onto everything and refuse to let some situations pass? Do we hold onto the past and try to draw our nourishment from that which no longer provides it? Are we not eliminating who or what is no longer beneficial? Are we not taking time to assimilate new experiences? Do we not approve of ourselves and so do not see what life is offering us? Do we need to learn that there is time and space for everything we want to do?

Kidneys

The kidneys are glandular organs that excrete urine. They serve as filters of blood plasma to separate substances not needed by the body from those that are.

Kidney problems often reflect lack of discernment and discrimination. Our judgment may be off. Are we not recognizing who or what is or is not beneficial in our life? Are we not recognizing the good in our life? Are we not seeing that there is good and potential learning in all situations? Are we being too critical of ourselves or others? Are we wallowing in disappointment and failures and not using them to grow by? Are we approaching everything and everyone with rose-colored glasses, seeing only good in all things?

Knees and Elbows

All joints, such as knees and elbows, provide opportunity for ease of movement and use of limbs. They enable us to move and change directions in movements and activities. They are symbols of our flexibility and our ability to flow and move.

If we are having problems with joints, we should ask ourselves if we are being too stubborn and inflexible. Are we hesitant to try new things or new approaches? Are we hesitant to step out into new directions? Are the new directions in which we are moving too painful or unbalanced for us? Are we refusing to give in, or are there others around us who refuse to give in, whether right or wrong? Are we unforgiving of ourselves or others because of movements we have taken in the past? Are we unwilling to reach and stretch for new heights and new goals?

Legs

Our legs enable us to move in all directions. They are the symbols of the pillars of balance that must be kept in regards to all movements in life. They represent our ability to progress and evolve and to lift ourselves higher.

With legs, we have our feet on the ground and our heads in the sky. We are like trees. When we have problems with them, we should ask ourselves questions and examine what is going on in our life. Are we feeling unbalanced in some new areas of our life? Are we resisting movement? Are we resisting change? Are we blocking others from moving forward? Are we allowing others to block us? Are we afraid of the future and so stand immersed in the present or even the past? Are we hypocritical, saying one thing but doing another? Are we feeling insecure in our present space and time?

Liver

The liver is a glandular organ in the body that secretes bile, which contains bile salts. These bile salts have a detergent action, breaking down and cleaning (detoxifying) the blood so that the kidney can filter it into that which is to be eliminated and that which is to be re-absorbed as nutrients. It also functions with the immune system of the body.

Problems with the liver often reflect strong negative emotions that have not been dealt with by the individual. (Hence the significance of the phrase "eating at my liver.") Deep anger and chronic fault-finding—with yourself or others—can help weaken liver function. Are we trying to deceive ourselves about something negative in our life? Are we refusing to clean up an aspect of our life? Are we exposed to constant complaining and criticism? Do we have feelings of "I never do anything right"? Are we refusing to clean up the past and move on? Are we wallowing in self-pity and hatred? Are we not doing what we can to help ourselves? Are we refusing to take the initiative? (After all, the liver strongly affects overall metabolism.)

Lungs

The lungs are the respiratory organs of the body. They enable the exchange of gases, internal and external. The taking in of oxygen and the exhalation of carbon dioxide is the external function. The internal is the absorption of oxygen at the cellular level.

Breath has always had great significance attached to it in all societies on a mystical level. It is the assimilation of power and life. Inhalation and exhalation are the processes of involution and evolution—the integration of life and spirit.

Problems with breathing can reflect an inability on some level to take in and express life and energy. Are we feeling smothered or stifled in some area? Are we smothering or stifling others? Are we not feeling the right or not being allowed to live or participate in some aspect of life? Are we being made to feel this way? Is there suppressed crying occurring (often reflected in asthma with the trapping of air)?

Are we feeling trapped? Is there inflammation in areas that are our basic life breath, i.e., family, home, etc.? Are we not living life as fully as we could? Are we not feeling cherished and welcomed in our life settings?

Mouth and Teeth

The mouth is a powerful symbol. It is the point at which digestion begins in the body. It is also our center for speech, the ability to express and communicate. The teeth also aid in the breaking down of food in the initial stages of digestion, and they facilitate clarity of speech.

Problems with the mouth and teeth should raise any number of questions and possibilities. Are we not taking in that which is nourishing? Are we feeding on garbage and trying to sustain ourselves with it? Are we spending too much time chewing on things and not making decisions or taking action? Are we allowing what others say to eat at us (often causing teeth problems)? Are we chewing on ourselves for what we did not say? Is there a need to be more careful about what we say and to whom? Are we letting the words of others (their opinions) set our own? Are we refusing to express ourselves creatively? Are we grinding on that which we should let pass?

Neck and Shoulders

The neck is the point of connection between the head and the trunk, the upper and the lower. It and the shoulders are the bridge between the two. Bridges of every form have had great significance and symbolism associated with them. They enable us to cross over and to open to new realms. We can travel back and forth across them. Because of this, necks and shoulders often reflect flexibility in thoughts and perceptions.

If we are having neck and shoulder problems, we need to question ourselves. Are we being too inflexible in our thoughts? Are we being too rigid? Are we afraid to see what's on either side of us or behind us? Are we taking too much responsibility upon our shoulders? Are we taking responsibility for that which is not ours? Do we refuse to see others' points of view or perspectives? Do we allow others' refusals to see our perspective affect us?

Nose

The nose is that part of the body that helps cleanse and warm the air that we breathe, so that it can more easily be absorbed by the body through the lungs. It is through it that we also have the sense of smell. It is a symbol for recognizing ourselves and others, and the efforts of both, in an appropriate manner and from a correct perspective. It can be a symbol for setting boundaries.

The nose is very symbolic as well. It is a symbol of our intuition and our higher sense of discrimination and discernment. If we are having problems, we should be asking ourselves some questions. Are we feeling unrecognized? Are we not recognizing others in our life appropriately? Are we "putting our nose into other people's business" when we shouldn't? Are we allowing others to put their noses in our business inappropriately? Are we not recognizing the efforts and energy we should be applying to our daily activities?

Pancreas

The pancreas is a gland that secretes digestive fluids and the hormone insulin, which regulates the metabolism of glucose in the body. It works for the breaking down and conversion of our food into one of three groups—carbohydrates, fats, and proteins.

The pancreas is a symbol of not only our ability to discern the sweetness in our life, but to separate all elements and find ways of assimilating them. It is a symbol of converting all experiences into learning. If we are having problems with the pancreas, we should do some self-examination. Are we not finding time to enjoy the "sweeter things" of life? Are we refusing to see that there is something beneficial that can come from all situations? Are we frustrated with our life, unable to find sweetness or benefit to it? Are we angry with ourselves or are feeling rejected by life? Do we not approve of ourselves or feel we may not deserve some sweetness? Have we failed to realize that the bitter and the sweet both serve functions in our life? Is everything all work and no play?

Sex Organs

The sex organs are the center for our basic creative life force—the serpent fire of the kundalini. This is the primal energy of life, creativity, birth, healing, etc. It can be likened to the primal energy that lies hidden within the DNA spiral.

In the Western world we have lost a lot of the mysticism of these organs. The sexual drive is our creative life force. Anything we do—in any area of life—draws upon that most primal energy. The male organs often symbolize the activating force, while the female symbolize the formative or receptive force.

Problems with these organs should have us examining not only our attitudes of sexuality, but also how we express or do not express our own innate creativity. Do you accept and approve of all that you feel? Do you accept and enjoy being the sex you are? Do you have anger at your partner, mate, or spouse? Are you not expressing any creativity in your life? Is your creativity stifled? Do you have conflicting thoughts of your own sexual needs and desires? Are you allowing others (including society) to determine your sexual behavior? Do you have intimate support in your life or is it absent? Do you have difficulty with intimacy?

Sinuses

The sinuses are the air-filled cavities of the head. These cavities warm and moisten the air we breathe and they also serve as sounding chambers for the voice, adding resonance to it.

If we are having difficulty with the sinuses, are we allowing others to irritate us? Is what we have within our life aggravating and creating disharmony? Are we having difficulty with people close to us not listening to us? Are our words causing friction and irritation? Are the words of others (especially those closest to us) causing friction and irritation to us? Is our life becoming congested with others who either do not hear us or do not help us to make life smoother? Are others critical of us? Are we critical of others? Are we being overly critical of ourselves?

Skin

The skin is the outer covering of the body. It is the largest sense organ. It protects and is a sensory system itself. It is a symbol of our sensitivity and our self-worth. It is also a symbol of birth and rebirth, as the cells of the skin are continually regenerating.

Problems of the skin should cause us to do some strong self-examination. Are we being overly sensitive to situations in our life? Are others being insensitive to us? Are we "out of touch"? Are we not feeling good about ourselves at the moment? Do we dislike ourselves or where we are at this moment in our lives? Are we feeling unloved and unlovable? Are we afraid of being hurt? Are we trying to deaden our senses to outside influences? Are we taking responsibility for who, what, and where we are? Is our individuality being threatened? Do we need to be more protective of ourselves? Are we feeling confined and constricted?

Stomach

The stomach is the primary organ for storing, diluting, and digesting food. It is our reservoir. It is a symbol of the thoughts, ideas, and inspirations that we can learn to digest and assimilate. It is the reservoir from which we can draw to experience the new and open new worlds.

Stomach problems often reflect outer problems in digesting life's experiences. Are we afraid of digesting or experiencing the new? Are we holding onto that which is no longer beneficial or nourishing to us? Do we have fears of not being good enough "eating away" at us? Do we have difficulty digesting that we are good enough just as we are? Do we not approve of ourselves? Are we having difficulty assimilating new ideas, concepts, and perspectives, and putting them in motion in our life?

Throat

The throat is that part of the body that is comprised partly of the esophagus, the pharynx, the larynx, the trachea, and the tonsils. It is our canal for swallowing, for breathing, and for speech.

In general, the throat is a symbol of what we can swallow and what we can express. It is tied to creativity. Throat problems in any area can reflect unexpressed anger, stifled creativity, and obstinate stubbornness (a refusal to change or even be a little flexible). It can also reflect a continual speaking with criticism, venom, and/or anger. It can reflect an angry attitude of "When is it my turn?"

Problems in the throat area should be examined in relation to the specific area. The larynx, for example, is the voice box, but it also aids in swallowing. If this is the problem area, are we having trouble swallowing what is being expressed to us? Are we stifling and swallowing our words when we should be speaking out? Are we expressing ourselves inappropriately? Are we afraid to speak up? Are others doing the speaking for you? Do you not feel free to speak of your desires, wishes, etc.?

Some Occult Significances of Major Systems in the Body

Once we have examined the symptom of the dis-ease and the body part(s) most affected by it, we should also examine the entire system to which that body part belongs. Although a symptom may reveal itself more strongly around a particular organ or body part, it is usually affecting us systemically.

Examine the function of the system and look for its occult significance. This can provide great insight into the root cause of a problem. This is especially important if we find that when disease does manifest, it does so most frequently through a particular system. For example, some individuals may find that when dis-ease does manifest, it usually affects the respiratory system. For others, it may be the digestive system. Identifying these patterns is crucial to true holistic health. The systemic problem pattern is often the one to which we have a greater predisposition. Thus we may need to take extra preventative care of that system.

The following are some of the major systems in the body, along with guidelines to begin to understand their hidden significance and influence in our life and our health.

Skeletal System

This system is composed of the bones and the minor cartilages. It helps to convert chemical energy into mechanical energy. The bones are the framework in the skeletal system and they function in the movement of the body. They support the soft tissue, protect vital organs, work with blood formation, and provide a reservoir of minerals.

Problems in this system should make us examine what we may or may not be protecting. In the case of broken bones, what organs is that bone protecting? And what is the significance of that organ? What are our longstanding feelings on support or lack of support in our life? What is wrong with the structure of our life?

Muscular System

Movement is primal to all living things. In the human body, muscles enable the movement of the body through space and the transport of nutrients through the body as well. We have cardiac muscles, we have skeletal muscles, and we have involuntary muscles. Which does the problem exist in? This will tell us much.

What kind of muscular problem are we experiencing? In the case of sprains, the joint has been moved too far. Are we trying to do more than we are capable of? Are we overextending our reach? With muscle strain, the muscle is simply overworked. Where are we overworked in life? Why must the body manifest a problem to get us to slow down and take time for ourselves? Remember that the symptom, the organ, and the system all need to be considered.

Digestive System

This system works for the conversion of food and beverages to nutrients and energy for use by the body in its various functions. Its major organs include the esophagus, the stomach, the intestines, the liver, the pancreas, and the gall bladder. Its primary functions are twofold: ingestion and absorption.

Any problem in any area of the digestive system should cause us to examine our own ingestive and absorption habits. What are we ingesting that we shouldn't? Or what should we be ingesting and aren't? Are we not absorbing the new ideas that we are exposing ourselves to? Are we not using what we have available to us in our life? Are we being wasteful?

Circulatory System

This system is comprised of three major aspects: the fluid to circulate nutrients (blood), a pump to circulate the fluids (the heart), and vessels to contain the fluid (arteries, capillaries, veins).

Problems in any area of the circulatory system usually stem from some lack of vitality for some area of our life. Problems with circulation almost always are tied to emotions that are allowed to circulate or flow too easily (no control) or are not being allowed to circulate. In the latter, they build internally, often creating high blood pressure. Are we becoming locked in the past and afraid to move on? Are we not resolving old emotional issues? Are we harboring an attitude of self-defeatism?

Respiratory System

The respiratory system works for the acquisition of oxygen and the elimination of carbon dioxide. It functions for the exchange of all gases throughout the body. Its major organs include the lungs, the larynx, the trachea, and the bronchial tube.

Respiration is essential for life. A problem in this area often centers around issues of a right to life. Do we feel we don't have the right to be living the life we are? Are we feeling guilty about how we are living our life? Are we not being allowed to live the life that is best for us? Are we suppressing our life expressions and emotions? Is there an equal exchange in the life process? Do we take in as much as we give out, or is it all one-sided?

Reproductive System

This system not only has to do with the reproduction of the human being, but it is also important to the replacement of damaged or dead cells in the body. It is our most creative essence and system. In the male, the organs include the penis, the testes, and the scrotum. In the female, it includes the ovaries, the uterus, the clitoris, the vagina, and the mammary glands.

Problems in the reproductive system reflect problems in regards to our ability to be creative and productive within our own life. Are we not seeing productivity in the right perspective? Are we taking time to involve ourselves in activities that are creative and fun, the kind that rejuvenate and regenerate us? Do we have problems with our sexuality and its expression? Are we unable to express it fully? Are we happy we are the sex we are?

Eliminative System

This system works for filtering and excretion. Its primary organs are the kidneys, the urinary bladder, and the bowels. Problems in this area have to do with anything we are having difficulty releasing.

Are we afraid to let go of the past? Are we holding onto anger? Are we unable to decide what is good for us and what isn't? Are we afraid to let go of someone or something? Is there a fear we may no longer be needed? Are we afraid of what the new may bring us so we cling to outworn ideas, attitudes, and traditions?

Nervous System

This is the system for communication and control. It works to integrate the activities of all organs. It stores information, and it gives each of us two qualities: (1) irritability, which is the capacity to respond to changes in internal and external environments and (2) conductivity, which enables us to transmit messages along the nerve fibers. It is comprised primarily of the brain, the spinal cord, and the peripheral nervous system.

Problems with the nervous system can come from various sources. Are we trying to integrate too many activities in our lives? Do we not have enough activities to keep us occupied? Are we overly sensitive to criticism by ourselves or others? Are we being overly critical to others? Are we not communicating our needs clearly? Are others not communicating to us? Are we closed to new possibilities in our lives?

The Endocrine System

This last system is one of the most important to the entire energy system of the body. The endocrine system involves the glandular functions of the body. The endocrine system and the nervous system work intimately together to integrate, correlate, and control all body processes. The glands secrete hormone directly into the bloodstream to excite or inhibit the functions of various organs and tissues. These glandular hormones are biochemical catalysts.

Any problem in the endocrine system should make us evaluate how we are responding to situations in our life. Are we overreacting to people and situations? Are we inhibited in our response to people and situations in our life? Are we responding to life inappropriately? We should examine our responses.

Much of the endocrine system and its effects upon the body are still not understood. It is an intricate system that, although treated separately, has an intimate connection to all of the other systems. Many of the glands are often treated in association with other systems of the body. For example, the gonads, ovaries, and mammary glands are often dealt with in connection to the reproductive system, although they are also part of the endocrine system as well. This emphasizes the holistic operation of all of the body's systems and organs.

The effects of the endocrine glands upon the body are widespread. No organ can escape its influence, as these glands facilitate all cells in performing their duties in varying speeds and capacities. They are also intimately connected to the functions of the chakras, and thus influence our subtle body energies. (Refer to discussions of the chakra system in chapter 3.)

There are many glands within the body. The major glands are the pituitary, the thyroid, the adrenals, the thymus, the pineal, and the ovaries and testicles. There are other hormone-secreting glands as well. These include the mammary glands, the pancreatic islets, the parathyroid, and the hypothalamus. Each works intimately with the others, although they do have their own individual activities as well. Studying their individual activities more closely will provide clarification as to what may be aggravating certain glandular conditions of the body. The following will provide a starting point.

The pituitary gland is a governor. It affects the activity of most of the other major glands. It affects the entire immune system as well. Problems with it often reflect issues dealing with how our life is being governed. Are others overactive within it? Are we not active enough in choosing and deciding what is best for us? Are others always making decisions for us or are we always making decisions for others? This gland reflects issues of control and the proper balance within it.

The thyroid is a gland that acts as the body's thermostat. It governs our metabolic rate. It is affected by and can reflect issues of proper expression. This gland is connected to the throat chakra, and hyperactivity is often a reflection of an imbalance. A sluggish metabolism can reflect that we are sluggish in using our creative expression. Are we not expressing ourselves and doing what we need and want to do? Are we not claiming our own power, or are we doing it in an inappropriate manner?

The adrenals are our glands for self-preservation and protection. They assist in the breakdown of protein foods for the body, but they also stimulate the metabolism in times of need and emergency. These are the glands of emergency. Adrenals that are over-taxed can reflect long-standing anxieties and worries. Are we refusing to care or respond to important issues in our life or in the lives of those closest to us? Are others not responding to our issues?

The thymus gland has an intimate connection to the immune system of the body. If we are having difficulty with repetitive illnesses and such, we should ask ourselves important questions. Are we feeling we are better, and thus more immune to the effects of our activities? Are we not recognizing that our actions on any level have repercussions? Are we involving ourselves in issues and problems that do not concern us? Are we infecting others with our thoughts and actions? Are we allowing others' thoughts and actions to affect and infect us? Have we lost our ability to find sweetness and benefit in life?

The pineal is closely related to the nervous system, although no nerve cells have been found in it. Thus, it is often symbolic of opening to awareness beyond normal physical perceptions. It also has ties to the sexual functions of growth—both physical and spiritual. Are we utilizing our mental and physical (sexual) energies appropriately? Are we not seeing what is right in front of us? Are we not honoring all of our energies, sexual and metaphysical, seeing all aspects of ourselves as spiritual? Are we not being sympathetic to others or are others not being sympathetic to us?

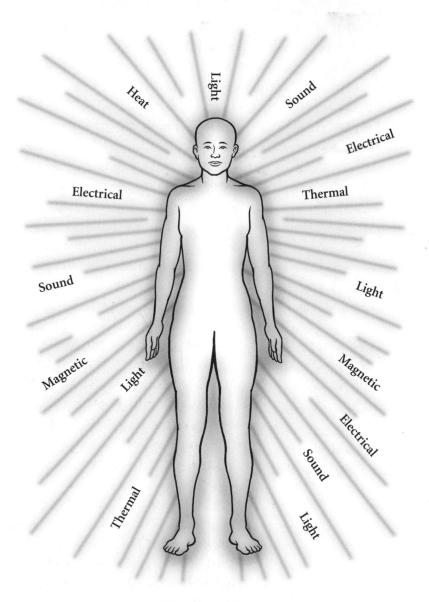

The Human Aura and Energy Emanations from the Body

There are a variety of energy fields that surround and emanate from the physical body. These include, but are not limited to, light, electrical, heat and thermal, sound, magnetic, and electromagnetic. These, along with the subtle bodies, comprise the entire aura and energy system of the human body.

three

VIBRATIONAL REMEDIES AND THE HUMAN ENERGY SYSTEM

The human body is an energy system. Both the ancients and the modern scientist agree that everything in life is formed of vibration. This vibration is the result of the movement of electrons and protons of every atom of every molecule of every substance. Vibration exists in objects, in animals, in people, and in the atmosphere around us. The vibrational frequencies of animate life are more active, vibrant, and variant than inanimate matter, but vibration exists in all.

The human body is comprised of many energy fields. These energy fields surround, emanate from, and can interact with the physical body and its various functions. These include, but are not limited to, light (colors), electrical, thermal (heat), sound, magnetic, and electromagnetic. One task of the holistic health practitioner is to determine which energies, intensities, and combinations are most effective in the healing process.

Surrounding the human body is an auric field. The aura is comprised of two aspects. This includes our subtle bodies, as described

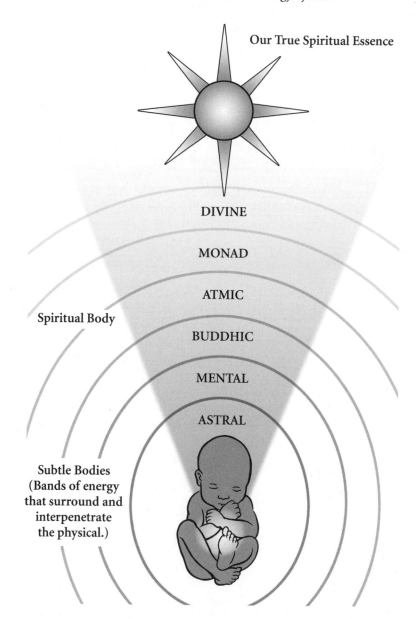

Our True Spiritual Essence

DIVINE

MONAD

ATMIC

Spiritual Body

BUDDHIC

MENTAL

ASTRAL

Subtle Bodies
(Bands of energy
that surround and
interpenetrate
the physical.)

The Formation of the Subtle Bodies in the Incarnation Process

Our true essence slows its vibrational intensity through stages so as to be able
to integrate with the physical vehicle without burning it up. These stages are
the subtle bodies, bands of energies that it molds around it, so as to more fully
integrate with the developing physical vehicle. The consciousness does connect
with the physical, though, from the moment of conception, but in increasing
intensity.

in traditional metaphysics, and it also includes the energy emanations of the human body itself.

The subtle bodies are bands of energy of varying intensity that surround and interpenetrate with the physical. Their predominant function is to help coordinate and regulate the soul's activities in the physical life. In Eastern philosophy, there are six subtle bodies surrounding the physical. Several Western traditions see them as four, with four of the subtle bodies being grouped generically as the spiritual body. (See the diagram on the previous page.)

For our purposes, we will focus on a four-body aspect of the human energy system: physical, astral (emotional), mental, and spiritual. For our greatest health, all four must be in alignment and harmonized. Psychological and physical problems result when there is a misalignment of the subtle bodies with the physical. This misalignment can be caused by trauma, stress, strong emotions, incorrect mental attitudes, etc. Thus we must work to have physical health, emotional health, mental health, and spiritual health.

An imbalance on any level will ultimately manifest itself in the physical, for it is the recipient of all subtle influences. It is through the physical that we must translate and express emotional, mental, and spiritual energies. It is through the physical that we live and experience life.

All of the organs, tissues, and systems within our body are comprised of similarly vibrating atoms. If something such as an allergen or contaminated food substance enters the body, it can alter the normal vibrational pattern of the body or a particular system. Along the same line, an unbalanced emotional or mental attitude can create a misalignment of the subtle bodies with the physical, altering the normal vibrational pattern of the body. At these times, the body needs something to help restore it to its original vibrational pattern. We can use vibrational remedies to temporarily restore balance to a problem area.

Vibrational remedies are subtle energy stimuli that interact with the energy systems of the human body to help stabilize and correct physical, emotional, mental, and spiritual conditions. By focusing the correct

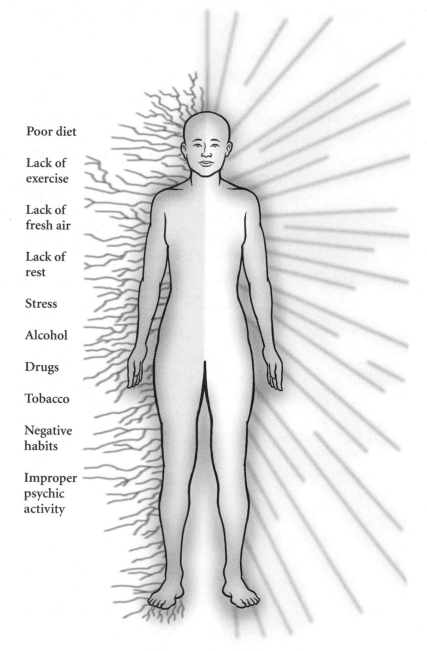

Poor diet

Lack of
exercise

Lack of
fresh air

Lack of
rest

Stress

Alcohol

Drugs

Tobacco

Negative
habits

Improper
psychic
activity

Weak and Strong Energy Fields

The stronger and more vibrant the aura is, the healthier we are, and the less likely we are to be influenced and impinged upon by outside forces.

vibrational remedy upon a problem area, we can temporarily restore balance to that area. When there is balance, the body is more effective in eliminating toxins and negativities that can hinder our body processes. Through vibrational remedies, we reinstill a proper flow of energy. Many times we fail to realize that the body knows how to take care of itself. Unfortunately, we do get in its way. We give it the wrong kinds of food. We overwork it. We don't allow it to rest. We expose it to stress and negativity. We hold onto emotions and attitudes that can short circuit its energy flow, causing weaknesses and imbalances.

Because the human body is an energy system, we can use various energy vibrations to interact with it. Some of the most common and effective vibrational remedies are sounds, colors, aromas, flower and gem elixirs, crystals and stones, and, of course, thought.

Vibrational Healing Through the Chakra System

Chakras[3] are the primary mediators of all energy within the body and coming into it. They mediate the electromagnetic and other subtle energy impulses of our energy system. They take our energy expressions and assist the body in distributing them for our various physical, emotional, mental, and spiritual functions.

Although not part of the physical body itself, they help link our subtle energy fields, surrounding and interpenetrating with the body to the activities of the body itself. Although often thought of as metaphysical "mumbo jumbo," modern science and technology are demonstrating that in the traditional locations given for the chakras, there is a greater emanation of electromagnetic energies from the body.

The chakras are connected to the functions of the physical body primarily through the endocrine glands and the spinal system. They mediate the energy within and outside of the body through the various

---

3 *Chakra* is a Sanskrit word meaning "wheel." It refers to a spinning vortex of energy that can be found emanating from predominant positions around the human body.

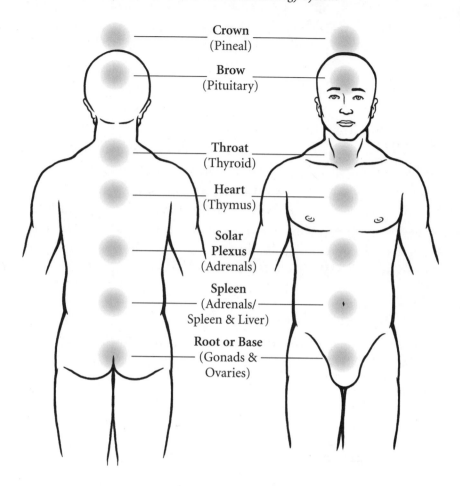

Crown
(Pineal)

Brow
(Pituitary)

Throat
(Thyroid)

Heart
(Thymus)

Solar
Plexus
(Adrenals)

Spleen
(Adrenals/
Spleen & Liver)

Root or Base
(Gonads &
Ovaries)

The Chakra System

The chakras mediate all energy within, coming into, and going out of the body. They help distribute energy for our physical, emotional, mental, and spiritual functions. The seven major chakras are points of greater electromagnetic activity within the auric field. The hands and feet are other points of great activity.

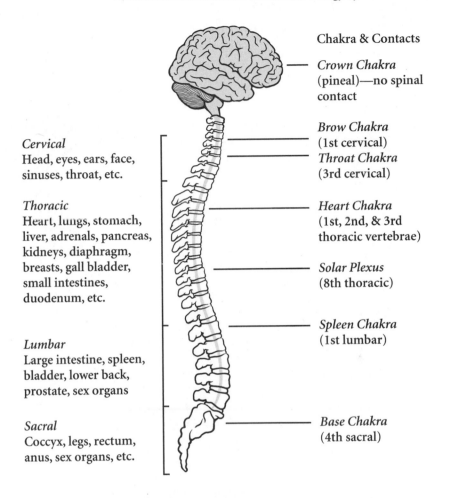

Chakra & Contacts

Crown Chakra
(pineal)—no spinal
contact

Brow Chakra
(1st cervical)

Throat Chakra
(3rd cervical)

Heart Chakra
(1st, 2nd, & 3rd
thoracic vertebrae)

Solar Plexus
(8th thoracic)

Spleen Chakra
(1st lumbar)

Base Chakra
(4th sacral)

Cervical
Head, eyes, ears, face,
sinuses, throat, etc.

Thoracic
Heart, lungs, stomach,
liver, adrenals, pancreas,
kidneys, diaphragm,
breasts, gall bladder,
small intestines,
duodenum, etc.

Lumbar
Large intestine, spleen,
bladder, lower back,
prostate, sex organs

Sacral
Coccyx, legs, rectum,
anus, sex organs, etc.

Spinal Contacts of the Chakras

Vibrations can be absorbed or projected through the chakras. This vibration is transmitted into the vertebrae of the spine, then transferred along nerve pathways to the organs, tissues, etc., to which they are linked. Imbalances can thus be balanced.

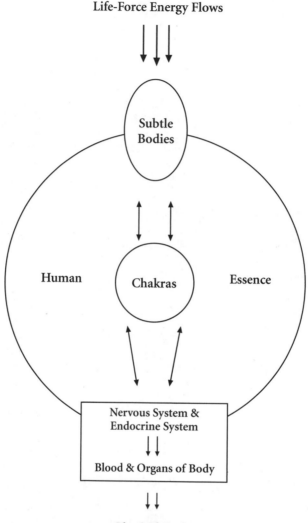

Life-Force Energy Flows

Subtle Bodies

Human   Chakras   Essence

Nervous System &
Endocrine System

Blood & Organs of Body

Physical Body

The Mediation of Energy Through Chakras

The normal life force from each subtle body enters into its own particular chakra, which then distributes the energy to the spinal contact, where it is in turn passed on to the blood stream and organs. When the food we eat is converted into energy, the process reverses itself so that the energy field and subtle bodies surrounding the physical are strengthened and energized for their own particular purposes.

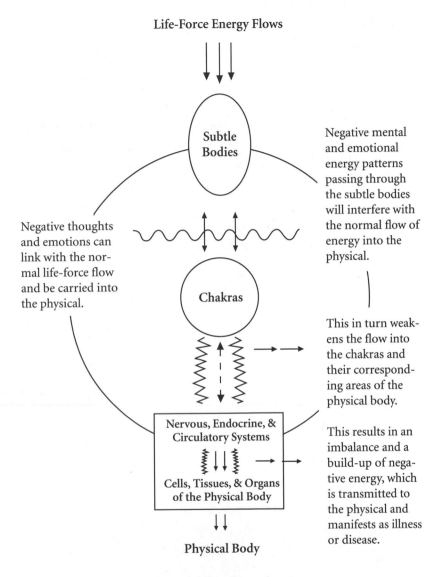

Blockage of the Flow of Energy

spinal contacts for distribution of energy through the body by means of the nerve pathways and the circulatory system. In this way, all of the organs, tissues, and cells receive the energy for their various uses.

At times of imbalance, the chakras attempt to pull greater energy and life force through the aura and the subtle bodies into the physical to counteract the dis-ease. If imbalances are not corrected, over time the chakras themselves may weaken and become unbalanced. They are then unable to draw energy in through the aura and subtle bodies. They may also become overactive, and thus create stress on various systems in the body. In either case, this is usually when a physical problem begins to manifest.

If we are to correct the condition, we must first restore balance to the subtle energy system and to the natural flow of energy to the physical. In many cases, simply restoring the proper balance and functioning of the chakras will either correct or alleviate the physical imbalance. Once the chakra energy flow is restored, the body itself can concentrate more fully on eliminating the physical expression of imbalance. The most effective means for restoring balance to the chakras, and thus to physical systems in the body, is through vibrational remedies. Such remedies may include sound, color, fragrance, etheric touch, crystals and gems, and even flower elixirs. Specific vibrations can be used to balance chakra activity, regardless of whether they are overactive or underactive.

Keep in mind that any imbalance within a person's energy field may reveal itself in physical, emotional, mental, and/or spiritual problems. Thus it is important to examine and understand both the metaphysical and the physical aspects of each chakra and their responses to vibration in any of its form. The rest of this chapter will delineate a number of these, and the rest of the book will begin to show you how to apply them for greater health within your life and other vibrations with which you may work.

The Base Chakra

Sacred Vibrations that Balance and Stimulate

- Tone of middle C

- Bass-toned and percussion instruments

- Long U vowel sound / Color red / Smoky quartz crystal / Sandal-wood and wisteria fragrances

Physical Effects

It is located at the area of the coccyx at the base of the spine. It is tied to the functions of the circulatory system, the reproductive system, and the functions of the lower extremities. It is our basic life-force center. It influences the activities of the testicles and ovaries, the legs and feet, and the pelvis area of the body.

Metaphysical Effects

This is our center for life-promoting energy. Stimulated properly, it can open awareness of past-life talents and ease fears. It is the seat of the kundalini within the body.

Emotional/Mental Attitudes Causing or Reflecting Dysfunction

Reactiveness; aggression, belligerence; manipulativeness; impulsiveness; recklessness; inability to recognize limits; abruptness; craving excitement; possessiveness and territoriality; needing approval; acting without thinking; power conscious; constantly active (hyperactivity); reluctance to defer gratification; bullying; obsessively sexual.

The Spleen Chakra

Sacred Vibrations that Balance and Stimulate

- Tone of D above middle C

- Bass-toned, percussion, brass, and woodwind instruments

• Long O vowel sound / Color orange / Carnelian agate / Patchouli and gardenia fragrances

Physical Effects

This center is tied to the function of the adrenal glands partially. It is also a major influence on the reproductive system and the entire muscular system of the body. It influences the eliminative system and the activities of the spleen, bladder, pancreas, and kidneys. It is a major center influencing the detoxification of the body.

Metaphysical Effects

This is a center influencing sensation and emotion. It is tied to the consciousness of creativity. It is a center that controls most personality functions, and it can be stimulated to open one to communication with energies and beings upon the astral plane.

Emotional/Mental Attitudes Causing or Reflecting Dysfunction

Selfishly arrogant; lustful; proud; conceited; vanity; the drive to belong conflicting with the desire to elbow one's way in; mistrust of others; following the crowd; worrying what others think; unable to get along with others; value social status; expansive without substance; power-seeking; antisocial.

The Solar Plexus Chakra

Sacred Vibrations that Balance and Stimulate

• Tone of E above middle C

• Flutes, woodwinds, strings, and piano instruments

• Vowel sound of "awh" / Color yellow / Citrine and topaz / Rosemary fragrance

Physical Effects

This center is linked to the solar plexus area of the physical body. This includes the digestive system, the adrenals, the stomach, the liver, and the gall bladder. It assists the body in its assimilation of nutrients. It is also linked to the functions of the left hemisphere of the brain. Many crippling diseases, ulcers, intestinal problems, and psychosomatic diseases are eased by working with this center.

Metaphysical Effects

This center is tied to the function of clairsentience and general psychic energies and experiences. It also has links to the rational thought processes. When activated for nonphysical purposes, it can reveal the talents and capacities of other souls. It can open the attunement to the influence of nature's elements within our lives.

Emotional/Mental Attitudes Causing or Reflecting Dysfunction

Feeling deprived of recognition; aloofness; dogmatic; fearing group power; isolation; confining life to a narrow view; always planning but never manifesting; constantly needing change and novelty; judgmental; critical; mentally bullying; feeling self is unerring; absolutist attitude.

The Heart Chakra

Sacred Vibrations that Balance and Stimulate

- Tone of F above middle C

- Harps, organs, flutes, wind chimes, and all string instruments

- Long A vowel sound / Colors green and pink / Rose quartz and tourmaline / Rose fragrance

Physical Effects

The heart chakra is influential in the function of the thymus gland and the entire immune system. It is tied to the functions of the heart itself and the circulatory system of the body.

It affects the assimilation of all nutrients and it is tied to all heart and childhood diseases. It is linked to the right hemisphere of the brain and its processes. It is also tied to the process of tissue regeneration.

Metaphysical Effects

This is the mediating center of the chakras. It is the center that awakens compassion and its expression in our lives. It is our center of higher love expression and healing energies. If stimulated properly, it opens sight of the deeper forces in plants and animals. It awakens knowledge of the sentiments and disposition of others as well.

Emotional/Mental Attitudes Causing or Reflecting Dysfunction

Anger; always expecting confirmation from others; unable to enforce will; financially insecure; emotionally insecure; uncertain; miserly; wanting to possess love; needing recognition from others; possessive; jealous and envious; self-doubting; always blaming others; mistrustful of life.

The Throat Chakra

Sacred Vibrations that Balance and Stimulate

- Tone of G above middle C

- Harps, organs, pianos, and high string instruments

- Short vowels (e, i, a, u) / Color blue / Turquoise stone / Bayberry and wisteria fragrances

Physical Effects

The throat chakra is tied to the functions of the throat, the esophagus, the mouth and teeth, the thyroid, and the parathyroid glands. It is influential in the functions of the respiratory system, and the functions of the bronchial and vocal apparatus. The alimentary canal is also part of its area of influence.

Metaphysical Effects

This center is tied to the functions of the right hemisphere of the brain and the creative functions of the mind. It can be stimulated to open one to clairaudience and to manifest greater abundance within our lives. It can be stimulated so as to survey the thoughts of others (telepathy), and it opens the consciousness to insight into the true laws of natural phenomena.

Emotional/Mental Attitudes Causing or Reflecting Dysfunction

Surrendering to superiors constantly; trapped by fixed ideas; clinging to tradition; always needing rules and supervision; rigidly dogmatic; resisting change; melancholy; fanatical; rigidity and stubbornness; authoritarian; being slow to respond.

The Brow Chakra

Sacred Vibrations that Balance and Stimulate

- Tone of A above middle C

- Harps, organs, pianos, wind chimes, and high string instruments

- Long E vowel sound / Color indigo / Lapis lazuli and fluorite / Eucalyptus fragrance

Physical Effects

The brow chakra influences the functions of the pituitary gland and the entire endocrine system of the body. It also has links to the immune system. It affects the synapses of the brain. It is a balancing center for the functions of the hemispheres of the brain. It is linked to the sinuses, eyes, ears, and the face in general.

Metaphysical Effects

This is the center for higher clairvoyance and the entire magnetism of the body (the feminine aspects of our energies). It opens one to higher and clearer perceptions. It is intricate in the process of the imagination and creative visualization. It can open one to spiritual vision.

Emotional/Mental Attitudes Causing or Reflecting Dysfunction

Worries; fear of the unconscious; fascination with external intelligence; pursuing idolized relationships; impatience; lateness for appointments; superstitiousness; inefficiency; unable to live in the now; "spaced out"; forgetfulness; fear of the future; undisciplined; introverted; oversensitivity to impressions of others; unable to manifest.

The Crown Chakra

Sacred Vibrations that Balance and Stimulate

- Tone of B above middle C

- Harps, organs, pianos, wind chimes, and high string instruments

- Long E vowel sounds / Color violet / Amethyst / Frankincense and lilac fragrances

Physical Effects

The crown chakra is tied to the functions of the nervous system and the entire skeletal system of the body. It influences the pineal gland and all nerve pathways and electrical synapses within the body. It is also linked to the balanced functioning of the hemispheres of the brain.

Metaphysical Effects

This chakra is the link to our spiritual essence. It aligns us with the higher forces of the universe, and it is powerful in the purification of our subtle bodies in preparing them as separate vehicles of consciousness. It can open one to all past lives and how they have led to this point within the present incarnation. It is critical to integrating our spiritual self with our physical self within the circumstances of our present life.

Emotional/Mental Attitudes Causing or Reflecting Dysfunction

Feeling misunderstood; inability to have enduring relationships at deep levels; intense erotic imaginations; needing sympathy; feeling misunderstood, shame, self-denial, and self-abasement; negative self-image; daydreamy; need to feel popular or indispensable; not understanding need for tenderness.

part 2

VIBRATIONAL HEALING
THROUGH THE
SENSE OF TOUCH

four

ETHERIC TOUCH

M ost people only see or experience as much as is necessary or essential to them and their immediate lives. People today are ignorant of their bodies as an energy system. There often exists the attitude that "we have physicians, so why take the time ourselves?" Thus we give over our responsibilities and a lot of our innate power and control over our health. When we are so casual about our own physical body and its energies, it is no wonder there is such strong prejudice about the more subtle energies of life.

We can develop the ability to experience the more subtle energies of life tangibly. We can learn to recognize that our energies do not stop at skin level. Our hands are points in the body with greater sensitivity. We can develop this sensitivity to feel subtle energy emanations from the body, as well as project them into the body.

This ability to project healing energies through the hands is known by many names. In more ancient times, it was called the "king's touch." Some today call it "therapeutic touch," while others simply call it the "laying on of hands." For our purposes, we will call it "etheric touch." It is a method of using the hands to direct energies (human and spiritual) to help heal.

Through our hands we will learn not only to sense energy imbalances around and in the body, but also project vibrations to help restore balance. We learn to use our hands as a catalyst to stimulate the other individual into healing him- or herself.

This form of vibrational healing is most effective for alleviating pain and aches and for general relaxation. If you bump your elbow or scrape your knee, what is usually the first thing you do? Place a hand on it and hold it. It helps alleviate the discomfort. Our hands are natural tools for healing, and everyone has the ability to develop it even further.

Unfortunately, when it comes to healing through such a subtle technique, we are often dealing with a person's belief system. Regardless of tangible results or scientific verification, if a belief is held that no such thing is possible, the task of opening to its realization can be difficult. Most people grow up with little or no acknowledgement of the subtle energies of life. Any such experiences are often attributed to "coincidence" or an overactive imagination. The exercises and techniques that follow in the rest of this chapter will assist you in breaking down any limiting thoughts or ideas you may personally hold. They will increase your sensitivity.

Results will vary from individual to individual. Persistence is the key, as everyone can experience tangible results. Initially, some of the exercises may be more successful than others. Do not be discouraged at any failure during initial attempts to experience the subtle energies through the hands. As with any ability, it takes time and practice. The ability to use etheric touch has lain dormant for many years. We must begin to stretch those unused abilities slowly and persistently. If you persist, you will succeed!

Remember that learning to use etheric touch is a commitment to yourself and to others. Approach the exercises with sincerity and keep in mind that you are embarking on a lifelong process of self-improvement. You are initiating a process that will enable you to know yourself and others more intimately. You are stepping out into areas of sacred perception.

To enhance your development, practice with a partner, so that you can get objective feedback. Also learn the ability of relaxed concentration. Trying too hard can block your progress. Learn to meditate and relax the body before the exercises. Perform a short, progressive relaxation. Take a few moments, close your eyes, and breathe deeply from the diaphragm. Focus on each part of the body individually, starting at your feet and working your way to the top of your head. Mentally send warm, relaxing feelings into that area of the body. See it, feel it, imagine it.

The more relaxed you are, the better your concentration will be. The more relaxed you are, the more sensitive you become to the subtle energies you are encountering and working with. Relaxation creates a hyperaesthetic condition. You become hypersensitive. If you have ever been jarred from a reverie or daydream by a phone ringing or a loud noise, you have experienced one aspect of this condition.

When we are relaxed—in an altered state of consciousness—we experience outside energies more intensely. A phone ringing will seem louder. Smells are stronger; light and colors are brighter. Touch is more sensitive. Because of this, relaxation assists us in perceiving and directing energies with the hands more effectively.

EXERCISE 1   *Feeling and Experiencing Our Subtle Energies*

In this exercise we are simply working to become more sensitive to the subtle emanations surrounding the physical body. This exercise can be performed by yourself, but you can also adapt it to practicing with a friend.

1. Begin by taking a seated position and performing a general, progressive relaxation.

2. Rub the palms of the hands together briskly for about fifteen to thirty seconds. Our hands are strong points of sensitivity and we do have minor chakra centers in them. This rubbing helps stimulate the chakras in the hands, increasing their overall sensitivity.

3. Extend your hands about a foot to a foot and a half in front of you, the palms facing each other. Hold the hands about two feet apart.

4. Slowly move the hands toward each other. Bring them as close to each other as you can without touching them.

5. Draw them slowly back to about six inches apart. Repeat this slow, in-and-out movement. Keep your movements slow, steady, and deliberate.

6. As you perform this exercise, pay attention to what your hands are feeling or sensing. You may experience a feeling of pressure building. There may be other sensations. There can be a sense of rubberiness, tickling, or a thickness building between the hands. You may experience warmth or coolness. You may even experience a pulsating sensation.

7. Take a few minutes to try and define what you are feeling. Do not worry about whether you are imagining it or not. Do not worry that it may feel different than what others experience. That is okay. Remember that we each have our own unique energy system, and so we each may experience the sensation differently as well. You are working to develop your own subtle perceptions.

8. This exercise assists in developing concentration. It also assists in helping you to recognize that our energy fields do not stop at skin level. You may wish to record in a notebook your impressions and experiences with this exercise, so that you can compare it later with what you experience as you develop further. This will help you to recognize your progress in experiencing subtle energies.

9. Once you have completed the above exercise, you will want to take it a step further. Bare your weaker arm. Hold your dominant hand about a foot above the bare arm.

Feeling and Experiencing Subtle Energies

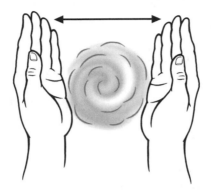

The in-and-out movement of the hands causes the energy surrounding them to accumulate between them, making it more perceptible to us. The hands are becoming more sensitive to the subtle energies.

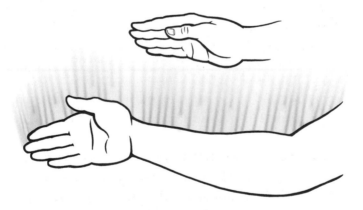

As the hands become more sensitive, we can use them to detect the auric energies emanating from other parts of the body as well. These detections may feel like heat, pressure, tingling, etc.

10. Slowly lower your hand toward the bare arm. Pay attention to anything that you might feel. How close do you come to the forearm before you feel the energy from it? Remember that the feeling may be one of pressure, thickness, coolness, warmth, tingling, etc. It will feel much like what you experienced between the hands. It may not be as strong, but you should be able to feel it. If you cannot, slowly repeat the exercise. Remember that we are reawakening our ability to be consciously aware of the subtle energies around us.

EXERCISE 2   *Sending and Feeling Energy Patterns*

An old occult axiom states "All energy follows thought." Wherever our thoughts are focused, so are our energy patterns. Our energy adjusts itself in accordance with our thoughts. We tell ourselves we will get two colds every winter, and the body's systems begin to work and adjust so that we are more susceptible to catching those two colds.

We go through a wide variety of thoughts and emotions on a daily basis, and those we are repeatedly exposed to or expressing will affect our energies. Exposure to outside energies also can impinge upon our energy fields and affect overall balance. These energies can be anything from anger and lust to pressure to buy. They can be energies of warmth and friendship or those of manipulation. The more sensitive we become to our energy fields, the more we can recognize and control what is allowed to affect them.

In the following exercise, we are working to increase our awareness of how outside energies can impact us. As we increase our sensitivity, we can learn to block the negative and restore healthy energy patterns. We can learn to heal.

1. Make yourself comfortable in a seated position. Take a few minutes to relax. You may wish to keep your eyes closed during this exercise, but it is not necessary.

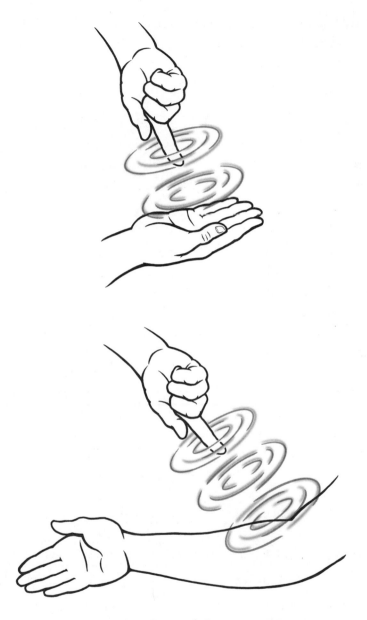

Sending and Feeling Subtle Energy Patterns

2. Hold one hand palm upward. Point the index finger of your other hand into the palm of the first. The finger should be three to six inches away from the other hand.

3. Take slow, deep breaths. As you breathe in and out, imagine the energy building and accumulating in the hand with the pointed index finger.

4. After several minutes of this, slowly begin to rotate your index finger in a small circle. Visualize a stream of energy spiraling out from the index finger to create a circle of energy that touches the palm of the open hand. Don't worry about whether you are imagining it or not, as we are working to prove that energy does follow thought.

5. Pay attention to what you feel within the palm of the hand. Just as in the previous exercise, the feeling may vary from person to person. You may feel a circle of warmth forming. A thickness, pressure, or tingling in the form of a small circle within the palm of the hand may also be experienced. Sometimes closing your eyes at this point can help you feel the sensation more strongly. The more you project and focus the energy with your mind, the stronger the sensation will become.

6. Having worked with the palm of the hand, next perform this exercise upon a naked forearm. Visualize and send the energy out through the finger in spirals of energy to impact upon the forearm. Pay attention to what you feel. With time and practice, the kind of sensation you experience will remain much the same, but its intensity will increase. Through exercises such as this, you begin to train yourself to recognize those feelings which let you know when something is impacting upon your energy field.

7. A powerful variation of this can be practiced with a partner. It is especially important for when we begin to use etheric

touch in healing. Have the other person stand with his/her back to you. Hold your hand(s) about six to twelve inches from your partner's back, palm open and facing the back.

Begin slow, rhythmic breathing. As you breathe in, feel the energy being drawn through your body and into the hand(s). As you breathe out, visualize and imagine the energy pouring through your hand(s) to the back of your partner. Slowly move the hand(s) in a simple geometric pattern—a circle, a square, a triangle, etc. Draw this energy pattern on your partner's back with the energy you are directing through your hand(s). Know in your mind that it is being felt by the individual.

Concentrate as you project the energies. Sometimes visualizing the stream of energy as a warm red light will help the partner to sense it more tangibly. Don't be afraid to experiment.

8. Have your partner try and identify the energy shape being drawn upon them. Pay attention to what they describe and experience. Compare it to what you discovered through the other exercises. What are the similarities? What are the differences? What can you do, or did you do, to make the feelings more intense and identifiable? Switch places and allow your partner to draw patterns on you. Compare the similarities and differences.

9. Gradually increase the distance. How far can you stand from your partner and still experience the energy pattern? Does it feel differently when the distances are extended? Pay attention to the responses. This increases your overall sensitivity to subtle energies and their effects upon you.

10. Experiment with this. Visualize colors streaming from your hands or fingers. (Refer to chapter 7 on color therapy for further guides.) Which colors are experienced more distinctly? Place different fragrances on your hands. (Refer to

the chapters on aromatherapy.) Are the experiences intensified? What happens when you tone and visualize the tone vibrations flowing through your hands? Learn which method or methods can be used by you personally to amplify your sensitivity to subtle energies and your ability to direct them consciously.

EXERCISE 3   *Increasing Hand Sensitivity*

Our hands can easily sense energy changes and differences. We have all experienced some aspects of this. When we touch someone or shake their hand, we get definite impressions about them. Our sense of touch helps us to attune to that individual's energy.

One of the most effective ways of developing and testing your hand sensitivity is through the use of color flashcards. The true effects and power of color will be covered in greater detail in later chapters. For now, though, we will use colors to increase our sensitivity. Remember that every color is an expression of energy and has its own unique qualities and characteristics.

1. Take a set of 3 x 5 index cards and on one side color it using a marker, crayon, etc. Use one card for each color. On the other side, you can list some of the qualities of the color. Begin with just the rainbow colors of red, orange, yellow, green, blue, indigo, and violet.

2. Relax the mind. Perform a progressive relaxation. Take a moment to study the cards singly. Focus on the color, and then read the characteristics to yourself.

3. With eyes closed, shuffle and mix the colored cards. Make sure that the colored surface of the cards are facing upward. Pull one from the set, and hold either one or both hands over it. Stay relaxed. Allow your hand to do the sensing. Does it have a warm feel or a cool feel? If warm, it is in the red and orange spectrum. If cool, it is in the blue spectrum.

Developing Sensitivity of Hands

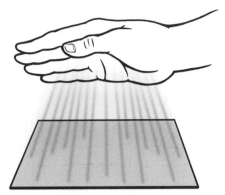

Developing a sensitivity to color through touch.

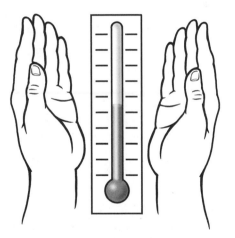

As we learn to radiate energy through our hands, we can change temperature through projecting color; red to warm, blue to cool.

4. What else do you feel or sense as you hold your hand over the colored card? Do you think you know what color it may be? Is there any kind of tingling? Do you notice anything in any particular part of your body? Pay attention to every impression, no matter how odd it may seem. These little details will eventually help you in becoming more knowledgeable of the color and its possible effects and applications.

5. With practice you will be able to identify color by its feel. Remember that you are working with subtle vibrational energies. You are working to develop your sensitivity to the subtle energy fields surrounding you.

EXERCISE 4   *Increasing Your Ability to Project Energy*

Through this exercise we learn that we can project energies through our hands. Remember: "All energy follows thought." Where we put our thoughts, that is where our energy goes. If we focus on a color, the energy emanations from the body begin to change to a frequency that resonates with that color. To demonstrate this, you will need an everyday outdoor thermometer.

1. Begin by taking a few moments to relax and focus your thoughts.

2. Bring your attention to your hands and rub them briskly together for fifteen to thirty seconds. This activates the chakras and increases their sensitivity.

3. Now take the thermometer and place it between your hands. You may either hold it in your hands or place it so that your hands are two to three inches from both sides of it.

4. Begin slow, rhythmic breathing. As you breathe slowly in, see and feel your body filling with a bright, warm, red energy. Try to imagine it as fire. Visualize it gathering in your hands. As you exhale, see and feel this hot energy pouring out of your hands toward the thermometer. Visualize, imagine, sense, and

project. Imagine it as red heat that streams from your hands to impact upon the thermometer. Continue this for three to five minutes. See how much you can raise the temperature of the thermometer.

5. Draw your hands away and visualize them and your body returning to normal. Allow the thermometer to return to room temperature as well.

6. Now begin your rhythmic breathing again. As you inhale, see and feel yourself filling with a cool, icy blue energy. See it gathering at your hands. As you exhale, visualize this icy blue energy streaming forth from them to impact upon the thermometer. Imagine, see, and feel your hands sending streams of icy energy like a cold north wind. See how much you can lower the temperature in three to five minutes.

7. Have fun with this exercise, and practice it frequently. This shows you concretely that you can direct and alter the energy emanations from your hands by your thoughts. You are learning to project energy vibrations of varying frequencies.

Performing Etheric Touch

Through the previous exercises we demonstrated that our energy does not stop at skin level, and that our hands can become sensitive to the subtle energy fields surrounding the human body. We also demonstrated that we can radiate energy outward from our hands by breathing and a concentration of thought.

Healing through etheric touch is working with the subtle energies surrounding the physical body. It is a form of healing that does not depend on actual physical contact with the human body, although sometimes it can be enhanced by it. (One example of this is explored in the next chapter on working with meridian therapy.)

This form of healing has always been considered more of a spiritual form. Unfortunately, when you mention that you do spiritual healing, many assume that it is healing based solely on faith and the healer's alignment with some divine force. Although etheric touch can be enhanced by that, its effectiveness is not dependent upon faith or the divine. (Unless one recognizes that the divine operates within each of us and is accessible by each of us.)

How the healing process actually takes place is still poorly understood. Even so, it is important to acknowledge that when we perform certain acts, specific effects will result. We all have the capability of effecting changes in our energies, physical and subtle, even if we don't understand it all. The ability is innate within us all. What we must discover and develop are the techniques that enable us to awaken and channel it for our various purposes.

Keep in mind that healing always comes from within. It is the individual who heals him- or herself. You may be the catalyst, and an assistant to boost the individual's own recuperative system, but the healing comes from within.

Before you being to work with anyone, know what you are going to do. Understand the process. Understand the metaphysical causes of physical dis-ease. Make no claims. Explain how our energy system operates. Perform some muscle testing, as described later in this book, to prove the metaphysics of energy.

Never work with another person if you are tired or ill. Although it is true that when we work to heal another we in turn are healed and balanced, working with another while we demonstrate illness ourselves can set up mental blocks and hinder the receptivity of the healing energy.

There are two steps to performing etheric touch. The first is using your hand sensitivity to assess possible problem areas. (Remember that you cannot diagnose unless you are a medical doctor. All you can do is describe your impressions of energy fluctuations in the field of an individual.) The second is directing the energy to effect a healing or balancing.

The assessment helps us to recognize where imbalances are within the energy field of an individual—physical or subtle. Any imbalances within the physical body will be reflected by imbalances in the subtle energy surrounding the body. This may be detected as a change in temperature, a difference in feel (more pressure or a mushiness), etc. The key in the assessment is to recognize changes or differences, no matter how subtle they may seem to be.

The healing is the projection of specific or general energies to correct imbalances. This may include directing energy through specific chakras and their physiological systems. It may also include sending general healing vibrations throughout the entire body. Each individual will differ, and you must develop a trust and flexibility in your effectiveness to work with another's energy. This comes with time and practice.

1. Always begin by centering yourself. Relax. Do a progressive relaxation or meditation prior to starting.

2. The individual may either sit, stand, or recline in front of you. Whatever is most comfortable for you and the individual is what will work best. Rub your hands briskly together for fifteen to thirty seconds to activate the chakras in the palms of the hands.

3. Begin with the front side of the individual to be healed. Place your hand about three to six inches from the person's skin. It does not matter where you begin, although it often seems more natural to begin at the top of the head and work your way to the feet. Begin with either side of the body and draw your hands slowly down, moving over each area of the body. Note anything you experience or may even imagine that you experience. Don't discuss them as you notice them. Just make a mental note and continue. Take about ten to fifteen seconds for each area of the body.

4. Allow your hands to scan the entire front of the body and then repeat with the back of the body. Again, note any differences and any impressions.

5. When you have completely scanned the entire body, go back and double-check any area you were not sure about.

6. Then take a few minutes and discuss with the individual what you experienced, where you found changes in the feel. Don't be afraid to ask for feedback or information on possible problems associated with those areas. This is how you get confirmation in what you are sensing with your hands and develop trust in it.

7. Some possible guidelines for interpretation of what you experience are:

   a. Warmth or hot spot = an inflamed area or overactive (overenergized) area. This can also reflect an area of the body in which there is a chronic problem or a recent acute problem. It can also sometimes indicate a point in the body in which stress is manifesting as a physical imbalance.

   b. Thickness or heaviness in pressure = an area of greater congestion. It can indicate a blockage or hindrance in the flow of energy or operation within an organ or system in the body. It can sometimes indicate an area of greater sensitivity, in that the body will sometimes pad an area in the aura with extra energy to protect it.

   c. Coolness = often reflects a blockage in a flow of energy within a system or to a particular organ or area of the body. It can reflect poor circulation and movement in some area of the energy system. It often reflects congestion.

8. Now we begin to balance out the energy field and project healing vibrations through the hands to the problem areas. Begin rhythmic breathing. Exhaling audibly will increase the flow of energy through you. Focus your mind on energy pouring out through your hands to correct and heal the condition. As you inhale, see and feel yourself filling with uni-

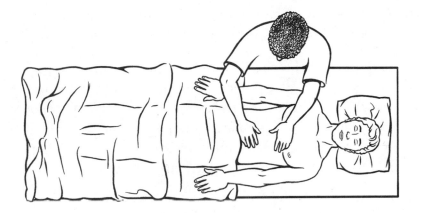

Healing Through Touch

You are becoming a channel of healing energy. As you breathe, you pull energy down through you and radiate it out your hands to heal and balance the individual. The energy takes on the frequency of your thoughts and focus. As you concentrate on a particular color, the radiations take that frequency, and the color is absorbed by the person being treated. The process heals and balances, and it awakens your high intuition and sensitivities.

versal healing energy. You may visualize it as a color or in any form you desire. As you exhale, visualize the energy streaming forth to cleanse, balance, and heal the problem area, along with the entire system to which it is associated.

9. Next move to the chakra(s) to which the problem area is associated. For example, if there is a stomach upset, begin by working on that area of the stomach. Next visualize the entire digestive system being balanced and healed. Then move your hands and attention to the solar plexus chakra, which mediates energies of the digestive system and stomach. Project balancing and strengthening energy to the chakra.

10. Now move to the base chakra area. Radiate energy through you to energize and strengthen it. Do this for several minutes. Then repeat this with each of the seven major chakras. Visualizing the energy in the appropriate color for each

chakra can enhance the process. This balances the entire
chakra system, and it strengthens the entire healing process.

To conclude the healing, move to the head area and project crystalline energy through you and into the individual. See and feel it
pouring out and filling the entire being of the individual. Visualize it
radiating in and around them with strength and vibrancy.

Remember that it is not your personal energy you are using in
this healing technique. As you perform rhythmic breathing, you are
drawing universal energy through you and projecting it to the other
individual.

five

THE MIRACLE OF MERIDIANS

The ancient oriental approach to true health is extremely holistic. The entire principle of healing elaborated in the text *The Yellow Emperor's Classic of Internal Medicine* by Ilza Veith is based on restoring balance. It recognizes that everything influences everything else. There is an intrinsic interaction and an extrinsic interaction involved in health. Intrinsic interaction is the intimate relationship between all organs and operations within the body. The extrinsic interaction is the intimate relationship with the environment of the individual. Neither should be excluded when working with health.

The Chinese recognized two energy sources. The first is that which is termed *iei*, or energy created through the elements of food and other nourishments we take into the body and which flow through the bloodstream. The second is *chi*, which is the universal life-force energy that flows through meridians.

Chi circulates through the body along well-established channels that join points of energy. The patterns of these channels are called meridians. Meridians are closely associated with the nerve pathways of the autonomic nervous system, which in turn is linked to every organ and part of the body. Learning to quiet, balance, and stimulate these channels of energy thereby affects all organs and parts of the body as well.

This life force circulates throughout the entire body in a twenty-four hour period. Each meridian and the various organs affected by it have an approximate two-hour influence by chi. The energy moves from one meridian to the next, thereby circulating this life force to all parts of the body. In essence, we are an energy system of perpetual motion.

These channels of energy or meridians for chi are throughout the body. They have been measured and mapped, and can be physically felt. Also along these lines are specific electromagnetic points (those used in acupuncture and acupressure). The meridians are named for the organ or system with which they are most closely associated.

There are fourteen meridians. Twelve of these run on each side of the body and the remaining two are on the midline. Each meridian has a definite pathway on the body and a specific direction in which the energy flows on that pathway. It is because of this pathway that an acupuncturist can use the needles on the hand to cure a headache. The meridian is a conductor of the energy impulse generated by the needle. It transmits this impulse along the pathway to restore a proper flow of energy throughout it, thereby eliminating the headache.

Every meridian has a starting point and an ending point. The ending point of one meridian is linked to the beginning point of the next. Thus all the meridians are interconnected. There is an endless cycle of free-flowing energy. Imbalances—physical, emotional, mental, and spiritual—can hinder this flow of energy and eventually help create dis-ease.

A problem in an organ or a system may be caused by a problem in its corresponding meridian or vice versa. It may also be caused by a blockage or problem in the meridian(s) that precede it within the normal cycle of this energy flow. If we build a dam in a river, the points beyond the dam will dry up and a multitude of problems can occur. Thus the normal flow has to be reestablished in order to correct the problem area. A healthy body depends upon maintaining all of these energy channels and their free flow.

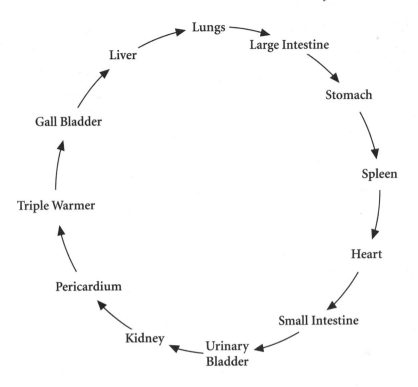

The Cycle of Chi Through the Body

A problem in one meridian and its corresponding organs could be caused by a blockage in the meridian preceding it. Thus breathing problems (Lung Meridian) may have their source in the Liver Meridian.

A primary concept of meridian therapy is polarity. All energy is governed by three polarities: positive/electrical (yang), the negative/magnetic (yin), and the neutral. That which is referred to as yin and yang are the electromagnetic polarities within the body that are intimately entwined. How these charges interact within our system determines how well the body functions and how we operate on a day-to-day basis.

Yin and yang are opposite forces in a single unit—opposing and complementing. They exist simultaneously, but under favorable conditions they can influence each other beneficially. Yang illnesses and problems can be cured or balanced by yin energy stimulation, and yin illnesses and problems can be overcome by yang.

Yang is the positive, active, and electrical aspect of chi within the body. Yin is the more passive, receptive, and magnetic aspect of chi in the body. As these charges interact, they determine how well our bodies function. Where there is balance, there is no restriction in the flow of energy and its operation; thus there are no problems with our health.

The yang energies expand upward and outward along the arms, legs, and body, and the yin energies contract downward, along the inside of the arms, legs, and body. Just as the planets revolve around the sun and the electrons and protons around the nucleus of the atom, so do the yin and yang meridians circulate around the central axis of the body.[4]

Two neutrally charged meridians flow through this central axis. These are called the Conception and Governing Meridians. The Conception Meridian governs the Lung, Spleen, Heart, Kidney, Pericardium, and Liver Meridians. The Governing Meridian governs the Large Intestine, Stomach, Small Intestine, Urinary Bladder, Triple Warmer, and Gall Bladder Meridians. (The specific functions and energies associated with each meridian will be explored later in this chapter, along with methods of working with them.)

Every yin meridian and its organs are paired with a yang meridian and its organs. The energies flow along one meridian until it reaches the end and then it flows along the path of the meridian to which it is paired. The pairs are as follows:

---

4 Quantum physics and the development of superconductors bring much light to this process. Any machine of perpetual motion normally has no freedom in movement because the electrons cannot pass freely. This creates friction, which can result in dis-ease and aging in the human machine. Meridian work, like superconductors, speeds up the activity of the electrons within the life force so that this energy flows freely throughout the body. This creates greater health and less opportunity for imbalance to occur.

Yin	Yang
Lungs	Large Intestine
Spleen	Stomach
Heart	Small Intestine
Kidney	Urinary Bladder
Pericardium	Triple Warmer
Liver	Gall Bladder

When working with meridian therapy, it is good not only to work with meridians most directly affecting the problem area, but also the one which immediately precedes the problem area, along with the paired opposite. Thus a problem in breathing may be corrected by working specifically with the Lung Meridian. It can also be helped by working with the Liver Meridian, as it precedes the Lung Meridian in the energy cycle. It may also be helped by working with the Large Intestine Meridian since it is the paired opposite of the Lung Meridian. It would help balance the polarity of the Lung Meridian.

Remember that the human essence is a holistic energy system. Everything affects everything else. We can not just treat symptoms. We must restore homeostasis and correct the problem's cause. This is what applying etheric touch to the meridians will enable you to do.

Practical Techniques of Meridian Therapy

EXERCISE 1   *Running the Meridians*

This exercise balances and restores the entire body metabolism to its natural rhythm and cycle. It is good to do this every morning or just once a week, and it is especially important to do it at any time there is an actual physical problem. It strengthens the energy system.

For this technique you can use either etheric touch or an actual physical touch. The physical touch can be made through slight pressure by the index finger. You may also run the meridians using a crystal or stone. Those that have been cut to have a rounded end serve very well in this capacity.

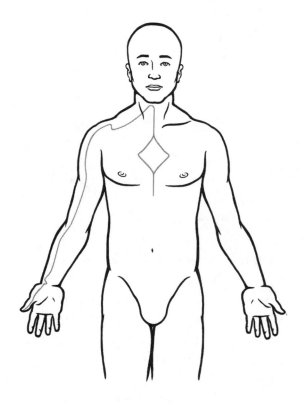

Lung Meridian

Location: Anterior aspect of the arm and forearm, ending near the thumbs
(chest, inner arm, and thumb tip)

Affects: Lungs, sense of smell, sinuses, mucous production, skin, sense of smell

Illnesses Reflecting Imbalance: Chronic cough, chest discomfort, breathing
difficulty, sore throat, fever, influenza, asthma, bronchitis, etc.

Polarity: Yin

Time of Day Most Active: 3:00–5:00 A.M.

Time of Year Most Critical: Autumn

Vibrational Therapies: White and soft blues / The long A (ay) sound and short
E (eh) sound / Pungent smells

Metaphysical Lesson: Letting go

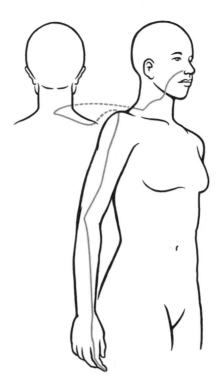

Large Intestine Meridian

Location: From the index finger, along the outer arm to the shoulder, the lateral border of the neck, and up to the bottom corner of the nose (outer arms, teeth, sinuses)

Affects: Intestines, sinuses, teeth, mucous production in digestion, the sense of smell, the nose

Illnesses Reflecting Imbalance: Abdominal pain, constipation, fever, toothache, diarrhea, and sore throat

Polarity: Yang

Time of Day Most Active: 5:00–7:00 A.M.

Time of Year Most Critical: Autumn

Vibrational Therapies: White and yellow / The "aw" sound and long E (ee) sound / Pungent smells (clove)

Metaphysical Lesson: Letting go

Stomach Meridian

Location: Below the eye, to the jaw line, around and back down to the neck, traversing the rib cage, down through the abdomen, along the anterior aspect of the leg and foot, ending at the second toe (face, chest, and outer legs)

Affects: Stomach, digestive system, vision, sense of taste, menstruation, knees, production of saliva

Illnesses Reflecting Imbalance: General intestinal distress, vomiting, stomachaches, facial paralysis, knee pain, gastritis, indigestion

Polarity: Yang

Time of Day Most Active: 7:00–9:00 A.M.

Time of Year Most Critical: Indian summer and humid times of the year

Vibrational Therapies: Color yellow / Sounds of "oh" and "ahh" / Sweet fragrances / Any vibrational method associated with the sense of taste

Metaphysical Lesson: Sympathy and reflection

Spleen Meridian

Location: Begins on the middle border of the big toe, ascends through the leg, thigh, abdomen, and lateral border of the rib cage and drops down to the axilla (inner legs, groin, and ribs)

Affects: Spleen, pancreas, menstruation, adrenals, groin area and organs, lower diaphragm, sense of taste

Illnesses Reflecting Imbalance: Gastritis, indigestion, abdominal distention, ulcers, vomiting, pain in the lower extremities, irregular menstrual cycle, impotence, anemia, generally run-down

Polarity: Yin

Time of Day Most Active: 9:00–11:00 A.M.

Time of Year Most Critical: Indian summer and humid times of the year

Vibrational Therapies: Orange-yellow shades of color / Sounds of "oh" / Fragrances that are sweet and minty

Metaphysical Lesson: Reflection and sympathy (overly abundant or lack of)

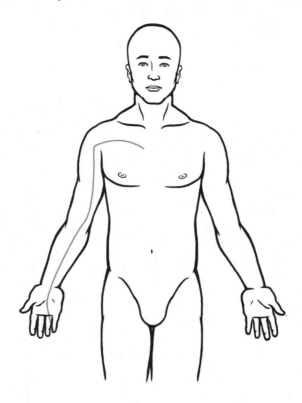

Heart Meridian

Location: Starts at the axilla and descends down middle border of arm, ending at the little finger of the hand

Affects: Heart, speech, shoulder, circulation, perspiration, and the tongue

Illnesses Reflecting Imbalance: Chest pain, palpitation, angina, jaundice, arm pain, cardiac disorders, insomnia, hysteria

Polarity: Yin

Time of Day Most Active: 11:00 A.M.–1:00 P.M.

Time of Year Most Critical: Summer

Vibrational Therapies: Colors of red, pink, or gold / The long A (ay) sound / Rose fragrance and bitter aromas

Metaphysical Lesson: Inner joy

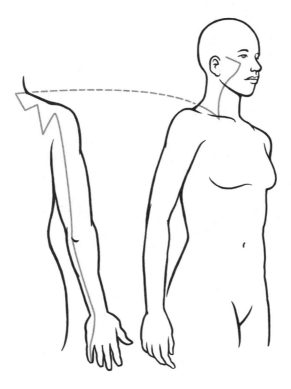

Small Intestine Meridian

Location: From little finger of hand, up the outer border of arm, with zigzags across the shoulder, neck, and up into face

Affects: Small intestine, lower abdomen, shoulders, throat, speech

Illnesses Reflecting Imbalance: Intestinal distress, shoulder pain, abdominal pain, earaches, tinnitus, tonsillitis, deafness

Polarity: Yang

Time of Day Most Active: 1:00–3:00 P.M.

Time of Year Most Critical: Summer and all hot times

Vibrational Therapies: Colors of red and blue/ Sounds of "aw" and long E (ee) / All bitter fragrances

Metaphysical Lesson: Inner joy

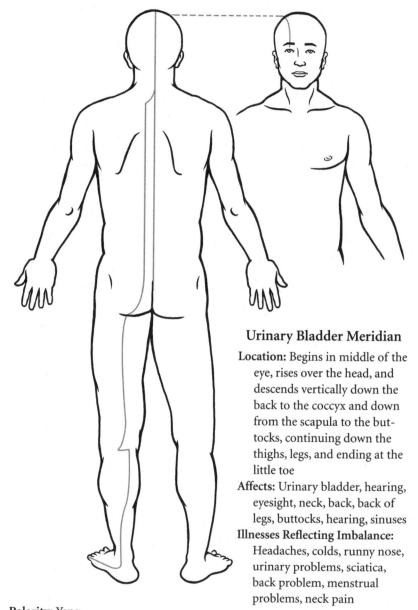

Urinary Bladder Meridian

Location: Begins in middle of the eye, rises over the head, and descends vertically down the back to the coccyx and down from the scapula to the buttocks, continuing down the thighs, legs, and ending at the little toe

Affects: Urinary bladder, hearing, eyesight, neck, back, back of legs, buttocks, hearing, sinuses

Illnesses Reflecting Imbalance: Headaches, colds, runny nose, urinary problems, sciatica, back problem, menstrual problems, neck pain

Polarity: Yang

Time of Day Most Active: 3:00–5:00 P.M.

Time of Year Most Critical: Winter and all cold times

Vibrational Therapies: Color black / Long U (oo) sounds and the musical scale / Lavender fragrance

Metaphysical Lesson: Overcoming fears and angers

Kidney Meridian

Location: Starts from the sole of the foot and ascends along the lateral aspect of the leg, through the thigh, abdomen, to the sternum, and ends at the clavicle area

Affects: Kidneys, bones, foot, inner legs, groin area, and the diaphragm

Illnesses Reflecting Imbalance: Kidney dysfunction, hypertension, constipation, loin pain, emphysema, irregular menstrual cycle, hiccups

Polarity: Yin

Time of Day Most Active: 5:00–7:00 P.M.

Time of Year Most Critical: Winter and all cold times

Vibrational Therapies: Colors of black and yellow / Sounds of long O (oh) and long U (oo) / Fragrances of mint and orange

Metaphysical Lesson: Clearing self of anger and fears

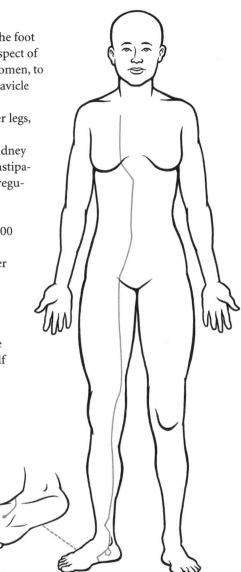

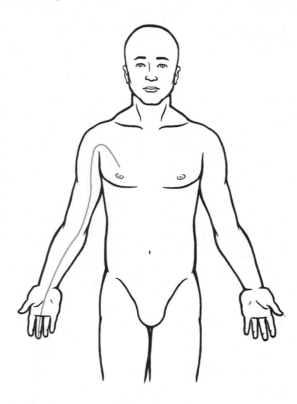

Pericardium Meridian

Location: Starts near the axilla, descends the anterior aspect of arm, and ends
at tip of the middle finger

Affects: Circulation, chest, growth, communication, heart

Illnesses Reflecting Imbalance: Chest pain, angina, drowsiness, coughing,
hand tremors, circulatory problems, heat stroke

Polarity: Yin

Time of Day Most Active: 7:00–9:00 P.M.

Time of Year Most Critical: Summer and all hot times

Vibrational Therapies: Colors of red and green / Sounds of long A(ay) / Flow-
ery and minty fragrances

Metaphysical Lesson: Growth through communication and relationships

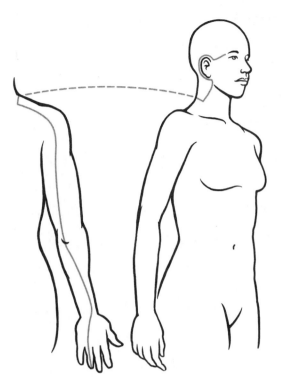

Triple Warmer Meridian

Location: Starts at ring finger, ascends along outer surface of arm to lateral border of neck, around the ears, and ends at edge of the eyebrow

Affects: Circulation, ears, temples, teeth, eyesight, face, and head

Illnesses Reflecting Imbalance: Headaches, sore throat, hearing problems, facial paralysis, toothaches, TMJ

Polarity: Yang

Time of Day Most Active: 9:00–11:00 P.M.

Time of Year Most Critical: Summer and all hot times

Vibrational Therapies: Color red / Tones of long A (ay) and long E(ee) / Fragrances of cinnamon, lavender, and clove

Metaphysical Lesson: Communication and growth in relationships

Gall Bladder Meridian

Location: Starts at the lateral border of the eye, travels the parietal and temporal region of the head, descends along the side of the chest, loin, and thigh to the foot, ending near fourth toe

Affects: Gall bladder, brain, sight, all organs and body parts on side of the body

Illnesses Reflecting Imbalance: Gall stones, headaches, migraines, vision problems, dizziness, stuffy nose, common cold, appendicitis, paralysis, hepatitis

Polarity: Yang

Time of Day Most Active: 11:00 P.M.–1:00 A.M.

Time of Year Most Critical: Spring and all windy times of the year

Vibrational Therapies: Color green / Sounds of long and short O ("oh" and "aw") / Sour fragrances

Metaphysical Lesson: Anger, decisions, and proper expression of will power

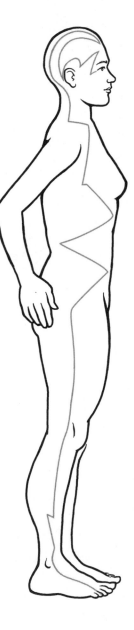

Liver Meridian

Location: Begins with the big toe, ascends through the foot and the inner side of the leg and abdomen, ending in mid-thorax at the beginning point of the Lung Meridian

Affects: Liver, the muscles, inner legs, groin, diaphragm, and ribs

Illnesses Reflecting Imbalance: Liver problem, hepatitis, abdominal pain, vomiting, pancreatitis, jaundice, irregular menstruation, hernia

Polarity: Yin

Time of Day Most Active: 1:00–3:00 A.M.

Time of Year Most Critical: Spring and most windy times of the year

Vibrational Therapies: Colors of green and blue-green / Sounds of long and short E (ee and eh) / Fragrances such as sage, carnation, and most sour aromas

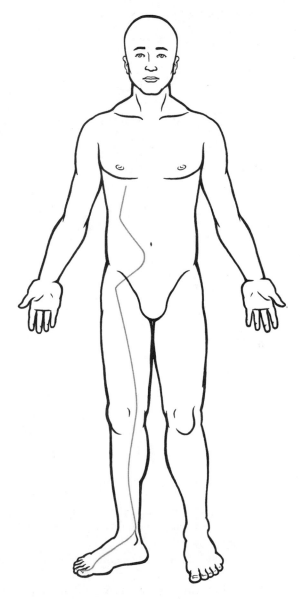

Metaphysical Lesson: Eliminating anger and proper expression of will power

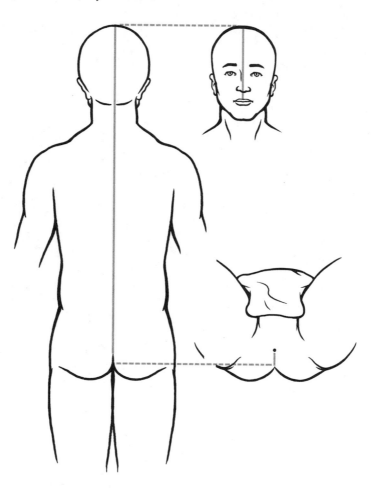

Governing Meridian

Location: Starts at the sacrum, travels up the spine, neck, over the head, down the face and nose to end at the upper lip, with an internal point just behind the upper front teeth

Affects: Spine, nervous system, skeletal system, anus and the sexual organs, and the brain and face

Illnesses Reflecting Imbalance: Nervous disorders, paralysis, sexual dysfunction, headaches, back pain, fever, mental disease, shock, and coma

Polarity: Neutral

Time of Day Most Active: All twenty-four hours

Time of Year Most Critical: All seasons

Vibrational Therapies: Colors of the rainbow / The tones of the musical scale / Fragrances affecting nervous system (lavender, eucalyptus, etc.)

Metaphysical Lesson: Ability to govern life or aspect of it

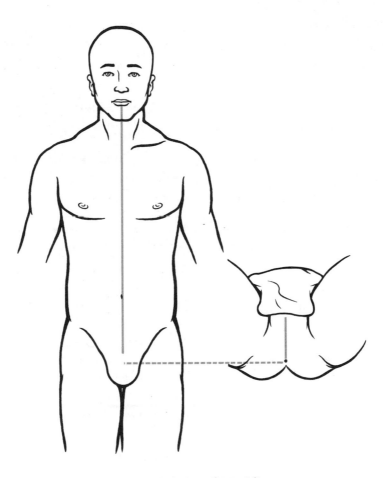

Conception Vessel Meridian

Location: Begins at the perineum between the anal orifice and the genitals, rises up midline in the front to a point at the tip of the tongue

Affects: Sexual organs, reproductive system, menstruation, male and female hormones, the circulatory system, and breath

Illnesses Reflecting Imbalance: Sexual dysfunction, hernia, reproductive problems, chest pain, problems of expression, esophagus problems, bronchitis

Polarity: Neutral

Time of Day Most Active: All twenty-four hours

Time of Year Most Critical: All seasons

Vibrational Therapies: Rainbow colors / The musical scale / Most flower fragrances, especially lilac

Metaphysical Lesson: Proper creative expression in all avenues

If extremely ill, tired, or stressed, your energy and its cycle is probably out of balance. Running the meridians will help restore homeostasis. This is also good if there is a chemical dependency. Any unusual chemical introduced into the body can confuse the body's communication system, thereby creating imbalances in the normal flow of energy throughout it.

1. Relax yourself. Do a progressive relaxation. Then begin rhythmic breathing. Visualize and know that as you do, energy is being drawn into you and can be projected through you.

2. Begin with the Lung Meridian. Hold your hands over one of its terminal points. As you breathe, see and feel energy pouring through you and out your hands to boost and balance the energy level of the meridian. Slowly move your hands along the pathway. Take your time in running the meridian. Trust what you feel, your own sensitivity, in deciding how quickly to move along it.

3. When you reach the other end of the meridian pathway, pause and then move your hands along it in the opposite direction. By running the meridians up and down, we are ensuring there are no blockages. Remember that with this exercise, we are simply trying to restore a balanced flow of energy throughout the body.

4. Then move to the next meridian and repeat the above procedure. Do this with all of them, in their proper order: Lung, Large Intestine, Stomach, Spleen, Heart, Small Intestine, Urinary Bladder, Kidney, Pericardium, Triple Warmer, Gall Bladder, and Liver. Refer to the chart on page 87.

5. Then move and do the same to the Governing and the Conception Meridians. Pause and send extra energy along these meridians at the points the seven chakras would be found along them.

6. If you wish, you may also simply trace the meridian along the surface of the skin with an index finger or a rounded edge of a crystal. This can create an even more tangible effect for the person being treated.

EXERCISE 2   *Detecting Problem Areas in the Meridians*

If you are having a particular health problem, the condition can easily be alleviated through simple meridian work. Pay attention to the times in which the symptoms manifest most frequently or most intensely. That will help you determine which meridian is either blocked or overly active. For example, if the condition is more aggravated around 2:00 in the morning, then there is probably an imbalance in the Liver Meridian, as that is the time of day it is most active. (Refer to the individual charts on each meridian.) Thus we know we need to give extra attention to the Liver Meridian when we are working on the body.

It is also a good idea to give extra attention to that meridian which precedes it in the cycle, as it is not unusual for the problem in one meridian to be intensified by a problem in the preceding. Remember the earlier analogy of the dam? Thus in this case, we would also give extra attention to the Gall Bladder Meridian as well.

1. After determining the specific problem meridian(s), perform your relaxation.

2. Begin the therapy by running the meridian(s) that are more specifically imbalanced. In the above example, we would begin by working with the Gall Bladder and the Liver Meridians. Use etheric touch on them, just as you have learned. This will help correct any specific problems in those specific pathways.

3. Then run the entire meridian cycle, beginning with the Lung Meridian as described in Exercise 1, "Running the Meridians," on page 89.

4. If you wish, you can then go back and give an extra boost of energy to the meridian(s) creating or manifesting the disease symptom.

5. Don't lock yourself into this procedure. Vary it according to the insights you receive while performing the etheric touch upon them. For example, you may wish to run the entire meridian cycle first and then concentrate on specific meridians that are creating imbalances. This can then be followed again by running the entire cycle again to reinforce and strengthen the flow of energy throughout the body.

EXERCISE 3   *Yin and Yang Meridian Work*

As described earlier, the meridians can be classified under different polarities. Except for the Governing and Conception Meridians, they can be classified as yin or yang (feminine or masculine). Yin meridians are paired with yang meridians. They balance and influence the operation of each other.

Many times an imbalance in a yin meridian (Lung, Spleen, Heart, Kidney, Pericardium, and Liver) can be corrected through its paired opposite, a yang meridian (Large Intestine, Stomach, Small Intestine, Urinary Bladder, Triple Warmer, Gall Bladder). Thus if you are having a problem in the Lung Meridian, you should also work with its opposite, the Large Intestine Meridian. If one is out of balance, its paired opposite will be as well. If one is overactive, the other will be underactive and vice versa.

1. Determine which meridian is out of balance and creating the physical symptoms you are experiencing. Then determine its paired opposite. (Refer to the chart on page 89.)

2. Relax and center yourself. Perform rhythmic breathing.

3. Apply etheric touch along the problem meridian, seeing it restored to balance. Then move to its paired opposite and apply etheric touch to it.

4. Conclude the therapy by running the entire meridian cycle.

EXERCISE 4   *Circulating Chi Through the Meridians*

This exercise involves the two neutral meridians. It helps to balance the polarities of the entire body. It balances and harmonizes the functions of the chakras and all organs and systems associated with them. It is strengthening to the overall energy and it alleviates stress.

This exercise can be performed by yourself. It is especially effective when performed outside and in the morning. It will circulate energy through all of the major organs and throughout the entire nervous system. It will give the cells in the body a boost to grow and to heal. It will open blockages and revitalize.

As seen earlier, the Governing Meridian runs up the back along the spine and over the top of the head. The Conception Meridian runs up the front of the body to the tongue. The two pathways can be connected through use of the tongue. It acts as a switch that connects the two currents of these meridians, creating an orbit of energy.

1. Take a seated position with feet flat on the floor and the back straight.

2. Center yourself. You may wish to perform a brief progressive relaxation.

3. Touch the tip of your tongue to the roof of your mouth, just behind the front teeth. This will link the governing and the conception meridians, creating a full circuit of energy.

4. Perform slow, rhythmic breathing. Inhale through your nose and exhale through your mouth.

5. Allow the energy to begin to loop in an orbit around the body through these two meridians. Consciously begin to direct it. As you inhale, feel the energy drawing upward along the spine. Feel it rise over the head and down the face. Feel it in the tongue, the throat, the chest, the navel, around the groin to the tailbone, and back up the spine again.

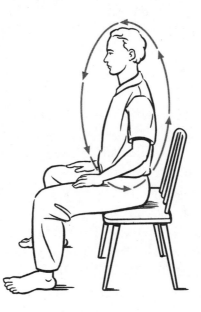

Position for Circulating Chi through the Meridians

6. Keep your breath slow and comfortable. Focus should be primarily on circulating the energy. Try and feel where the energy is moving at all times within this orbit.

7. You will begin to feel warm. This is a sign of increased energy circulation, a tangible clue. Continue for five to ten minutes.

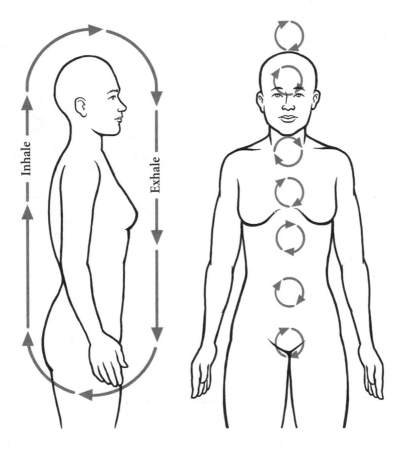

Breathing and the Microcosmic Orbit

Each circle of energy strengthens the chakra, causing stronger clockwise rotation and strengthening related physical energies. First perform rhythmic breathing to increase your energy. Then as you continue, feel the energy circulating up the spine and down the front. As it circulates, feel it energizing your chakra centers. You may even wish to see each orbit change to a different color, a color for each chakra.

part 3

VIBRATIONAL HEALING
THROUGH THE
SENSE OF SIGHT

six

THE MEANING AND POWER
OF COLOR

Color is a wondrous experience. It is joyful, and it affects us on multiple levels. Every color has the ability to touch us physically, emotionally, mentally, and spiritually. Some colors are warm; some are cool. Some soothe and others stimulate.

Often we hear of the divine or spiritual being described as light. This spiritual light that surrounds us and fills us is ultimately experienced and translated to us through the sense of sight. It is through vision that most people experience the essence of color, although some feel colors more dynamically and others even hear the subtle expressions of light that we call color. It is through color that we are able to experience the wonder of light.

Everyone is affected by colors, often more than they realize. Color is intimately tied to all aspects of our life, especially to its visual aspects. It permeates our language, our culture, and our health. We use colors to describe our physical well-being, our emotions, our attitudes, and our spiritual experiences:

"I'm in the pink today."

"He was red with anger."

"He was feeling a little blue after he lost."

"She was green with envy."

"It was a rich, golden experience."

No one is neutral when it comes to colors. There are some colors we like more than others, and there are some we do not like at all. At night we may pick out certain clothes for the next day, but we often discover upon awakening the next morning that they no longer are suitable or comfortable.

Did you ever wonder why this is so? The most common theory is that we are drawn to clothes with those colors that we most need at the time. When we pick out clothes the night before, we are choosing colors that we instinctively know would be beneficial for us at that time. After a night's sleep though, our energy system has changed. It is more rested and balanced, and the colors we had chosen are no longer suitable for the state we have awakened to.

We are drawn to those colors that we need. Often our responses are instinctive, but with practice we can become more conscious of the effects of color—physiologically or spiritually. How often have we been told that a certain color looks good on us? Have we said this to others? This reflects a sensitivity to color that we often ignore or do not pay enough attention to.

There are periods in our life where certain colors are more predominant within our wardrobes. There are times of the year in which we are drawn to and wear specific colors. Instinctively, we know what colors we need and when. We each have our own unique energy system and our own cycle of energy flow within our lives. We have to be careful about following trends in colors and begin following our own instincts in many regards. Then when we examine the physical and metaphysical effects of colors, it becomes easier to understand what patterns we are more likely manifesting or moving into within our life.

For example, some always seem to wear fall colors (darker, earthier tones) during autumn, and spring colors (the more pastel shades) in the springtime. They do not vary this, even when they feel a need for some spring colors during the autumn. Marketing strategists promote the idea of never wearing dark clothes during the spring and summer, except under special circumstances. If pressed for a rationale, you are likely to hear that the darker shades are insulating and too warm to wear during the hot summer months. And yet, there may be times in which wearing black during the spring and summer could be beneficial to you. You may need its energy to ground, insulate, and even give yourself a sense of peace in the midst of hectic activities. (Refer to the information on the color black given later in this chapter.) Does color truly affect us more than we realize? Can color be used to alter our physical, emotional, mental, and spiritual conditions?

The answer to both questions is "Yes," but we have to begin to pay attention to how we respond to color. Begin by asking yourself some simple questions:

- What is your favorite color?

- How do you feel when you wear that color, as opposed to other colors?

- Which colors always seem to strike you more strongly?

- Are there colors you do not like to wear?

- Are there colors that you do not like?

Keeping a color diary for a month or so can be very enlightening. Each day make a list of what colors you wore that day. At the end of the day, evaluate the day's activities. Try to wear the same colors at least two to three different times during the month. Then at the end of the month compare how the days went.

Were there certain days that were more productive? Hectic? Energizing? Depleting? What colors were you wearing on those days? Were there certain colors that you desired to wear more frequently?

Then begin to study the qualities of light and color. Examine some of the more esoteric aspects of color. You should be able to understand why you were drawn to and wore certain colors. The more you understand about color and light, the more you will begin to realize its subtle effects upon your life—from the clothes that you wear, to the color of your office, to the color of the car you drive, and more.

Remember that color is a property of light. When light is broken down into different wavelengths or frequencies, we end up with different colors. It is like holding up a prism to sunlight. As the light passes through the prism, it is broken into various vibrational frequencies, displaying a rainbow effect on an opposite surface. These rainbow colors are only a mere fraction of the entire light spectrum. There are multiple shades, and each has its own unique characteristics.

Every color, every frequency of light, has its own characteristics, and thus has a capability of affecting different energies of the human essence. Some colors, because they are of a higher frequency of the light wave, can affect the higher frequencies of the brain. Other colors, because they are of a lower frequency, can affect those systems or energies of the physical body which operates within it. The following chart gives an abbreviated look at the way certain light frequencies act upon our energy system, physically and otherwise:

Physical
Restful   = Green, light blue
Revitalizing = Orange
Stimulating = Red

Emotional
Restful   = Sky blue, turquoise
Revitalizing = Peach
Stimulating = Orange

Mental
Restful   = Indigo
Revitalizing = Emerald green
Stimulating = Yellow

Spiritual
Restful   = Blue
Revitalizing = Gold
Stimulating = Violet, purple

Color is a concentration of a certain light frequency. It can be stimulating or depressing, constructive or destructive. It can be repelling or attractive. Each color has its own unique effects and can be used for healing and balancing, as well as for stimulating deeper levels of consciousness.

Working with colors in healing involves two steps. First, you must understand the individual properties of each color. This will be explored in this chapter. Second, you must learn specific techniques to project and absorb color. These will be described in the following chapter.

To use color as a vibrational healing modality, you must become more color sensitive and knowledgeable. The more knowledgeable you become of light and colors, the easier you will find it to heal and balance with them. In my earlier book, *How to Heal with Color*, a number of exercises were described to facilitate sensitivity to color and light.

Within the realm of this book, we do not have time to explore them all, but there are several activities that you can do to develop greater sensitivity:

Play with Colors

In essence this means start exploring all the various shades of color. Go to a store and buy a 64-pack of Crayola Crayons. Most people grew up with these colors, and even to this day it is my reference for describing colors I see in auras or in healing work. Or, if you prefer, there are very inexpensive packs of colored pencils and markers that are now available.

Play with them. Draw with them. Buy a coloring book and color with them. Don't hold to the natural colors of objects. For example, if there are animals, make them whatever color you desire—even multiple colors. As you do this, pay attention to how you feel as you color. Which colors do you like the best? Doodle with them. Buy a paint-by-number set, but don't follow the numbers. Paint each section the colors you desire, no matter how out of the ordinary. Have fun with the process. Colors awaken a newfound sense of joy. You will be surprised how easy it is to slip into the coloring mode and lose track of time.

Create a Color Wheel

Take a sheet of paper and draw a large circle in the center. Then divide that circle into as many sections (at least twelve) as you wish. Color each section a different color. You may even wish to have a section for every color marker or crayon that you have. Do not color them in any particular order. You will find as you go along that you can easily recognize which colors seem to go better together. You are simply becoming more color aware.

Because this exercise employs so many colors, it also has other wonderful benefits. It will balance out your system and relax you. It restores balance to the chakras and to the subtle energy flows of the body, mind, and spirit. Make other smaller wheels, and combine just two or three colors. Pay attention to how they make you feel. Pay attention to your body, your emotions, and your mental states before, during, and after. You will be surprised at the effects.

The Meaning of Colors

The associations and uses for colors, as outlined below, are guidelines only. They are not inscribed in stone. They are characteristics to help you begin your own work with color therapy. As you work with each individual, you will discover that certain shades are more effective than others. You may also discover that certain colors may not work at all in regard to the individual's condition. Remember that everyone's energy system is unique unto itself.

In cases such as these, a little experimentation and a following of your own intuition will help you discover the best colors and combinations of colors for the most beneficial results. Keep in mind that the colors and their application must always be adapted to the individual.

When learning to apply the colors, keep in mind that the body and its chakras need all colors. The chakras often have a specific association with a particular color. This indicates that the chakra center may require a predominance of that color, but each chakra does need every color periodically. You are likely to find as you begin to explore color therapies that some chakras and their corresponding physiological systems may need a color other than the color normally attributed to it. Remember that we each have our own unique energy system and must adapt healing modalities to fit it. Often this is a trial-and-error process, until you are able to discover that method or combination of methods that works best for you individually.

Men and women also respond differently to colors. For example, when it comes to the color red, men are more drawn to and stimulated by the red-orange range. Women, on the other hand, are more drawn to reds in the red-violet range. Though men may not like pinks, women often find men who wear pink more appealing. Men and women who want to catch the eye of the opposite sex can wear the colors that will be responded to more strongly. As with all colors, there are effects beyond the physiological. Most bookstores and libraries have books on the psychology of colors, and these can be of great benefit when determining and using colors for therapeutic purposes.

White

Keynote: Purification, purity, amplification

Physical Applications: All systems of the body. White contains the entire light spectrum. It is strengthening. It is cleansing and purifying to the entire energy system. It can awaken greater creativity. When in doubt as to what color to use, you can seldom go wrong with white. It is also beneficial to begin and end a color therapy session with white to stabilize the energy system of the individual and to give it an overall boost. It amplifies the effects of any other color used with it in a healing session.

Black

Keynote: Protection, grounding, strengthening

Physical Applications: Effective in polarity therapy when combined with white. Black also contains the entire color spectrum within it. It is also a color that has had many confusing correspondences in the past. Many individuals shy away from using black in color therapy and healing, but I have found it to be beneficial at times. Black is a protective color. It is grounding and calming, especially to extremely sensitive individuals. It activates the magnetic or feminine energies of the body, strengthening them.

Black should be used sparingly, as too much black can cause depression or aggravate such emotional/mental conditions. Black is most effective when used in conjunction with white, balancing the polarities of the individual, especially in cases where the individual seems to be losing control. It can activate the subconscious mind, which can put life and all of its craziness into proper perspective. It should rarely be used by itself, but always in combination with another color.

The Rainbow Colors

RED

Keynote: Strengthening of the life force, will, and sexuality; stimulating

Physical Applications: Circulatory system, sexuality. Stimulating to the overall energy levels of the metabolism, lower extremities, most blood conditions. Red is a stimulating color. It will energize the base chakra. It warms and it activates. It awakens our physical life force. It can be used for colds, poor circulation, anemia, and mucous ailments. Red strengthens the physical energy and the will of the individual. It can stimulate deeper passions, whether they are of sex and love, courage, hatred, or even revenge.

Too much red can overstimulate and aggravate certain conditions. High blood pressure is an indication of too much red energy within the system. Red can be used to raise the body's temperature and to energize the blood. It is also balanced by the color green.

ORANGE

Keynote: Activation, construction, optimism, energy reserves

Physical Applications: Muscular system, eliminative system, emotional aggravation and causes of physical problems. Orange affects the second (spleen) chakra center. It is the color of joy and wisdom and creativity. It stimulates feelings of socialness. It is tied to our emotional health and the muscular system of the body. Too much orange affects the nerves, and it should be balanced with shades of green-blues. Orange can assist us in healing conditions of the spleen, pancreas, stomach, intestines, adrenals, food assimilation, and depression.

Individuals experiencing emotional paralysis can be helped with this color, especially the peach shades. Peach is a color that strengthens the aura and gives it a little extra cushioning in recovery processes. It and most shades of orange can be used to revitalize the physical body. It makes a good tonic after a bout of illness, for it is strengthening to the eliminative system of the body.

YELLOW

Keynote: Mental activity, intellectual power and ability, awakening

Physical Applications: Digestive system, gastro-intestinal tract, adrenal activity, left hemisphere brain activity. Yellow predominantly affects the solar plexus chakra, and it is stimulating to the mental faculties of the individual. It can be used for depression. It helps awaken an enthusiasm for life. It awakens greater confidence and optimism. It is also effective in the treatment of digestive problems. It is beneficial to the stomach, the intestines, the bladder, and the entire eliminative system as well. It is very effective in the treatment of most headaches. It helps to balance the gastrointestinal tract. The golden-yellow shades are healthful to both the body and the mind. It can be used to facilitate the learning capabilities of an individual.

Yellow is a color that catches the eye. It is one of the first colors that most people notice. It is also a color that can create or indicate anxiety and mental tension. Excessive amounts or exposures to it should be balanced with colors from the blue spectrum.

GREEN

Keynote: Balance, growth, calming

Physical Applications: Circulatory system, sympathetic nervous system, conditions aggravated by emotions. (Green should never be used to help heal tumorous or cancerous conditions, as green helps things grow.) Green is the most predominant color on the planet. It balances our energies, and it can be used to increase our sensitivity and compassion. It has a calming effect, especially in inflamed conditions of the body. It is soothing to the nervous system. The brighter greens, leaning toward the blue spectrum, are powerful in healing most conditions. Green can also be used to awaken greater friendliness, hope, faith, and peace. It is restful and revitalizing to overtaxed mental conditions.

Green strongly affects the heart chakra, and it is balancing to the autonomic nervous system. It can be applied beneficially in cardiac conditions, high blood pressure, ulcers, exhaustion, and headaches. It should never be used in cancerous or tumorous conditions, or with anything of a malignant nature, as green also stimulates growth.

BLUE

Keynote: Peace, faith, aspiration, creative expression

Physical Applications: Respiratory system, eyes, ears, nose, throat, venous conditions. Blue is cooling to the body's system. It is relaxing. It is quieting to our energies, and it has an antiseptic effect. It strengthens and balances the respiratory system. It is also excellent for high blood pressure and all conditions of the throat. It is beneficial to venous conditions of the body. Blue is very effective in easing all childhood diseases, along with asthma, chicken pox, jaundice, and rheumatism. It is one of the most universally healing colors for children.

Blue can also be used to awaken intuition and to ease loneliness. It is very effective when combined with the warmer colors in the orange and red-orange spectrum. It awakens artistic expression and inspiration.

INDIGO

Keynote: Integration, purification, altered states of consciousness

Physical Applications: Endocrine system, reproductive system, infection, most conditions of the head and face. Indigo and the deeper shades of blue are dynamic healing colors on both spiritual and physical levels. This color activates the brow chakra, and it is balancing to all conditions associated with it. It strengthens the lymph system, the glands, and the immune system of the body. It is an excellent blood purifier, and can be used to assist in detoxifying the body. It is a color that is also balancing to the hemisphere of the brain and all nerve synapses between them.

Indigo can be used effectively to treat all conditions of the face (including the eyes, ears, nose, mouth, and sinuses). Indigo also has a sedative effect, and it can be used in meditation to achieve deeper levels of consciousness. It can awaken devotion and intuition. It can be used for problems in the lungs and for removing obsessions. Too much indigo can cause depression and a sense of separateness from others. It can be balanced effectively with soft orange shades.

VIOLET

Keynote: Purification, transmutation, practical spirituality

Physical Applications: Skeletal system, nervous system, some venous conditions, cancerous/tumorous conditions. Violet is a color that affects the crown chakra. It also affects the entire skeletal and nervous systems of the body. It is very antiseptic, purifying on both physical and spiritual levels. It helps balance the physical and the spiritual energies. Violet is effective in cancerous conditions of the body. Arthritis can be eased by a violet light that leans more toward the blue shades. Violet also helps the body assimilate nutrients and minerals.

Violet also stimulates inspiration and humility. It assists in stimulating dream activity. In meditation, violet can help open us to our past lives, especially those that are presently affecting our health. A true violet is 50 percent blue and 50 percent red. It is the balance of the physical and the spiritual. It is a reminder that we need both aspects within our life for balanced health. Violet helps to restore a proper perspective both in regard to the mundane aspects of life (including the physical well-being), and the spiritual aspects, helping to keep them practical.

Other Healing Colors

AQUA (TURQUOISE AND OTHER LIGHT BLUE-GREENS)

Keynote: Multipurpose healing

Physical Applications: Respiratory system, strengthening to the metabolism. Aqua is cooling to the system. It can be beneficial in easing all feverish conditions and for balancing all systems of the body. It can also be used to cool and ease any inflammation. It combines both the beneficial effects of blue and green. It vitalizes all systems. It is also purifying. It can be used in treating skin conditions and throat problems, and it is very effective for acute pain and earaches. It eases respiration problems. It is effective in treatment of asthma and bronchitis, especially with children. Regular color breathing with aqua can prevent intense attacks of asthmatic conditions.

BLUE (ROYAL)

Keynote: Purifying

Physical Applications: It helps the body to assimilate oxygen. It assists in the exchange of gases, externally and internally. It can clear a foggy mind and it is an aid to negative physical conditions that affect the brain. It can help ease depression and emotional problems that can aggravate physiological conditions.

BROWN

Keynote: Grounding and stabilizing

Physical Applications: Brown is also an effective color in healing. It is especially effective in stabilizing overexcited states. It calms and grounds emotions and extreme mental conditions. Brown can help awaken common sense and discrimination. It brings us back down to earth. It is effective for any kind of spaciness. Brown, when it shows up in the human aura, can reflect a need for grounding. When it takes the shades of what I call "puke brown," it will often reflect infection in the body or that area of the body in which it overlays in the aura. Brown can be used to stabilize all systems. I have also found it effective to use in cases of hyperactivity with children, especially with combinations of colors in the rust to deep brown range.

GOLD

Keynote: Strengthening and amplifying

Physical Applications: Immune system, cardiac conditions. Gold is a color that can strengthen the energies associated with the entire immune system. It can be used with other colors to amplify the effects without overexciting the system. It is very strengthening to the heart. It is effective to use in regard to all cardiac problems, especially as a powerful tonic after heart surgery. Gold is a powerful stimulant to the immune system of the body. It helps awaken the individual's own healing abilities to assist the body in restoring homeostasis. It can also awaken renewed enthusiasm.

LEMON

Keynote: Mental stimulation

Physical Applications: Digestive system, left hemisphere brain activity. Lemon is vitalizing and stimulating to the brain. Thus it is effective in treating and alleviating conditions associated with it—i.e., Alzheimer's, senility, etc. It can be used to help stimulate the brain's natural abilities. It always has a shade of green within the spectrum, and in lemon, the green works as a cleanser. Lemons assist us in bringing toxins to the surface so they can be cleaned out. These may be physical toxins as well as emotional toxins. Lemon is also effective in treating digestive problems and appendicitis. It facilitates the natural digestive process, helping the body assimilate nutrients more effectively. Lemon is good for tissues and bones.

PINK

Keynote: Soothing

Physical Applications: Skin conditions and inflammations, immune system. Pink is a soothing color on all levels, physical and otherwise. Mentally and emotionally, it can be used to soothe conditions of anger and feelings of neglect. Pink can be used to awaken compassion, love, and purity. It can be used in meditation to discern greater truths. It is comforting to the emotional energies of the individual. Physically, pink is most effective in the treatment of skin problems and conditions, especially when combined with aqua. It also stimulates the thymus gland and eases stress upon the immune system of the body.

PURPLE

Keynote: Intense purification

Physical Applications: Detoxifying the body. Purple is considered by many to be a high vibrational color. It is this high vibration that gives it its ability for purification. It is effective to use when strong detoxifying of the body is needed, as in the case of cancerous or precancerous conditions. Purple is purifying to the body, but because of its high vibration, it should be used sparingly. Too much purple can create or aggravate depression. It can be used to stimulate venous activity in the body. It can also be used for headaches. The red-purple range is beneficial to balancing the polarities of the body. The blue-purple range is effective in helping to shrink (such as tumors) and to cool, easing inflammations.

SILVER

Keynote: Amplification and intuitive clarification

Physical Applications: Discernment of the cause of dis-ease. Silver can be used to amplify the effects of other colors, much in the manner of white. It is also effective in meditation, in discovering the metaphysical source of an illness or dis-ease. Unless we discover the source, the likelihood of its remanifestation is high. Silver can also be used to help discover and apply the creative imagination. It activates innate intuition. It is stimulating and balancing to the feminine energies, and especially the yin meridians.

Common Ailments and Their Beneficial Colors

This list is a guideline only. It is not prescriptive. It is a suggestion to help you find a starting point in working with color therapy. It is not designed to replace traditional medicine. Rather, it is to provide a means by which you can participate more personally in your own healing process. Use it as such, so that you can develop your own system of color application. Find what works for you. Remember that you may need to apply different colors with different intensities. Often, experimentation is the only way we have of discovering what works for the individual.

Begin all color treatment with white and end with white. This amplifies the effects and it serves to keep the color treatments from aggravating a condition. It provides balance. Remember that the red spectrum affects the physical and is stimulating and warming. Blues are cooling and cleansing, affecting the spiritual energies. The yellow shades serve to bridge them, affecting the mental energies. The three together provide opportunities for healing body, mind, and spirit.

Common Ailments and Their Beneficial Colors

Condition	Beneficial Colors
Abdominal Cramps	Yellow, Lemon
Abscesses	Blue, Blue-Violet
Aches (ear)	Turquoise
Aches (head)	Blue, Green
Aches (muscles)	Pastel Orange
Aches (tooth)	Blue, Blue-Violet
Acne	Pink, Red-Violet
AIDS	Red, Indigo, and Violet, followed by Pink and Gold
Alcoholism	Indigo, Yellow
Allergies	Indigo, Soft Orange
Alzheimer's	Royal Blue, Blue-Purple, followed by Yellow
Anemia	Red
Anxieties	Light Blue, Green
Appetite (excessive)	Indigo
Appetite (loss)	Yellow, Lemon
Arthritis	Violet, Blue-Violet
Asthma	Blue, Orange
Belching	Yellow, Lemon
Bladder	Yellow-Orange
Bleeding	Blue-Green
Blisters	Powder or Ice Blue
Blood Pressure (high)	Blue, Green
Blood Pressure (low)	Red, Red-Orange
Bones	Violet, Lemon
Bowels	Yellow-Orange
Breast	Pink, Red-Violet
Bronchitis	Blue, Blue-Green, Turquoise
Burns	Blue, Blue-Green
Cancer	Blue, Blue-Violet, followed by Pink

Common Ailments and Their Beneficial Colors (*continued*)

Condition	Beneficial Colors
Colds	Red
Diabetes	Violet
Eczema	Lemon
Epilepsy	Turquoise, Deep Blues
Eyes	Indigo, Royal Blue
Fevers	Blue
Growths	Violet, Blue-Violet
Hay Fever	Red-Orange
Heart Problems	Green and Pink
Hemorrhoids	Deep Blue
Indigestion	Yellow, Lemon
Infection	Violet
Inflammation	Blue
Influenza	Deep Blue, Turquoise, Violet
Kidneys	Yellow, Yellow-Orange
Leukemia	Violet
Liver	Blue and Yellow combinations
Menstrual Problems	Soft Reds and Blue-Green combinations
Nausea	Ice Blue
Nerves	Green, Blue-Greens
Parkinson's	Indigo
Pneumonia	Red and Red-Orange, combined with Indigo
Rash	Lemon and Turquoise
Skin Problems	Pink, Blue-Violet, Turquoise
Swelling	Pale and Ice Blues
Ulcers	Green

seven

SIMPLE COLOR THERAPIES

Identifying the color needed can sometimes be the easiest part of color therapy. Learning the methods of application, the length of application, and the right color combinations can be confusing, especially when it varies from individual to individual. The length of application will vary, depending upon the condition and the problem. Trust your own intuition and judgment, along with feedback from the individual. Start with five to ten minutes of a color at a time. This is almost always sufficient. For some, you may need to apply the color therapy over several sessions, either in the course of a day, a week, or longer. Be flexible on this.

As to the method of application, this also will vary. There are many methods of applying colors. Some color therapists use cloth swatches. Some wrap their clients in colored towels. Some teach their clients how to dress in colors for health. Some use colored lights, or even projectors with colored filters. Throughout the rest of this chapter are four color application techniques that any beginner or more advanced color therapists can use effectively:

- Rainbow visualization

- Applying color through etheric touch

- Performing color breathing

- Color therapy for the chakras

Do not limit yourself to these. Adapt them. Find which method or methods work most effectively for you.

COLOR TECHNIQUE 1   *Rainbow Visualization*

There are many variations for this exercise, so do not be afraid to adapt it. It is beneficial to do periodically, even daily. It is strengthening and healing to all systems and energies of the body, physically and spiritually.

1. Begin by taking a comfortable position, sitting or standing, whichever is more comfortable for you. Close your eyes and take three slow, deep breaths. When you exhale, see and feel all tension leaving the body.

2. Now in your mind's eye, visualize a rainbow that is arching over your head in the sky above. Now visualize a ball of red light spinning out of that rainbow down to the top of your head and into your body. Imagine it descending and spinning out vibrant red energy that touches and heals every part of your body.

3. Concentrate on this glowing crystalline energy. Allow it to spin down to your feet, filling you with its radiations. Then you can see yourself in that color. As it reaches your feet, the ball of red light dissipates and the red energy it left within you is absorbed by your body. As the last of the color is absorbed by the body, visualize an orange crystalline ball emanating from that rainbow overhead. Imagine it spinning down into your body, filling you in turn with vibrant orange energy from head to toe. As the ball of light reaches your feet, it dissipates, and the orange energy is absorbed into your body.

4. Continue this process with each of the remaining rainbow hues: yellow, green, blue, indigo, and violet. In turn, you fill the body with each color of the rainbow and allow it to be absorbed. As the last of the violet is absorbed into the body, see yourself shining with vibrant vitality and energy. See yourself balanced and healed. Then imagine the rainbow above you beginning to move, drawing down until it encircles you to become a permanent rainbow of protection and health surrounding your body. Know that each time you perform this exercise, the rainbow will grow stronger within you and around you. You will become more vibrant, healthy, and energized.

COLOR TECHNIQUE 2 *Applying Color Through Etheric Touch*

Just as we learned earlier that we could send energy through our hands, we can more effectively direct it by focusing and imaging a particular color of energy. Once you have determine the color necessary for the condition, the process of projecting it is simple:

1. Relax and center yourself.

2. Begin rhythmic breathing. As you do, visualize energy filling your body and gathering at your hands. Visualize this initially as a pure, crystalline white energy.

3. Just as you learned to do, project this energy throughout the individual's body to strengthen all systems.

4. Now pause briefly and shift your concentration to that of the healing color needed specifically for the individual's condition. As you continue your breathing, see and feel yourself filling with this energy.

5. As you inhale, draw this energy into you and as you exhale, visualize this energy streaming forth in the color you are focusing on. Remember that all energy follows thought. When we

focus upon a specific color, the energy we project through etheric touch takes on the frequency of that color.

6. Continue till you feel this problem is being balanced and healed. Then pause again and project through your hands that same pure crystalline white energy you used in the beginning. This will further strengthen the healing color you projected and further stabilize the body's health.

Sample Color Healing Through Etheric Touch

One of the most common ailments is the headache. It is also one of the easiest to eliminate through color. Most headaches are the result of an over-stimulation of the brow or crown chakra. This overactivity creates an "inflamed" kind of condition. Cooling these centers down serves to alleviate the problem most of the time.

For this exercise we will use etheric touch and the color of a soft, cool blue or a blue-green combination. For deeper pains, such as with migraines, projecting indigo can be effective. Take a few moments and relax yourself. Begin slow, comfortable, rhythmic breathing. As you breathe in, feel the universal blue energy drawing into your body and moving toward your hands.

Have the individual with the headache take a seated position in front of you. Instruct him/her to just close the eyes and relax. Place your hands two to three inches to the front and back of the individual's head. (See the picture on the following page.)

Continue your breathing. Now as you exhale, see and feel this cool blue energy streaming forth from your hands. Visualize it surrounding and permeating the head of the individual. Visualize it calming, soothing, and balancing the pain. Sometimes it helps to visualize the blue as a colored aspirin.

You may wish to move your hands to the sides of the head as well. The temple areas are often points at which energy blockage occurs, aggravating the headaches. Continue this for three to five minutes. Noticeable results rarely take any longer.

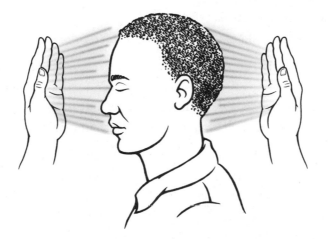

Healing a Headache with a Touch of Color

All energy follows thought. As we concentrate the mind on a particular color, that signal is sent to the energy being projected from the hands. The color we focus on determines the vibration of that projection. We can thus use our hands to heal or alleviate conditions through simple touch.

COLOR TECHNIQUE 3   *Color Breathing*

Proper breathing should always involve the diaphragm. Place your hands gently upon your navel. Inhale deeply. Do your hands move outward? Exhale slowly. Do your hands move back in? If so, you are breathing properly. Many people only breathe from the upper chest. In these cases, the air is not taken deeply into the body, and less energy and vitality is achieved from it.

On the less intricate side, performing color breathing (especially outdoors or by an open window) is a powerfully effective form of healing. Remember that air is turned into energy within the body. The frequency and strength of that energy is largely determined by our thoughts. Breathing different colors assists us with various health factors.

1. Make yourself comfortable. A seated position may be more comfortable, but make sure the spine is erect. Place the tip

of the tongue against the roof of the mouth, just behind the front teeth, to link the Conception and Governing Meridians.

2. Inhale slowly through the nostrils for a count of five or six. Then hold that breath for a count of ten to twelve. Then exhale slowly through the mouth for a count of five or six. Establish a slow, comfortable breathing rhythm.

3. Now as you breathe in, see and feel the air as a particular color. See and feel it filling your entire body. See and feel this color growing stronger within you with each breath. Visualize it balancing and healing whatever condition you wish to correct. Breathing this color for five to ten minutes can have wonderful effects.

4. If unsure as to the color, breathe in pure crystalline white light. You may also simply use the seven colors of the rainbow, balancing the chakras and energizing your overall system. Remember that different colors, even when breathed, will elicit different effects:

Red Breath

Energizing and warming. Helps with colds and sinuses. Drying to mucous membranes. Strengthening to overall energy levels. This can be a quick fix to alleviate cold and flu symptoms.

Pink Breath

Beneficial to all skin conditions. Good for puffiness. Eases anger and feelings of loneliness. It can be used to soothe most emotional and mental conditions.

Orange Breath

Balances the emotions. Healing to muscular conditions. Can help ease some respiratory problems. Awakens creativity. Restores joy for life. Orange and pink combinations (peach color) are especially good for

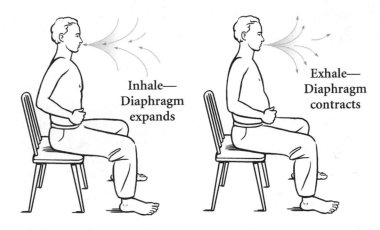

Inhale—
Diaphragm
expands

Exhale—
Diaphragm
contracts

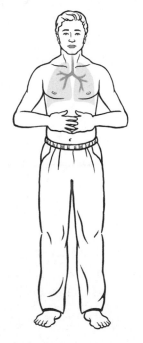

Proper Rhythmic Breathing

Inhale through the nose for a specified count. Hold the breath for the same count, and then exhale out the mouth for the count. You should be able to feel the diaphragm expand with each breath.

the muscles of the body. Peach breaths can also strengthen us so that we are less likely to be affected by uncomfortable environments.

Yellow Breath

Assists us in learning and assimilating information more easily and quickly. Eases indigestion and gas. The gold shade of yellow is an overall healing color and is beneficial in breath work for inner head problems.

Green Breath

Eases nervous conditions. Awakens greater sense of prosperity. Pale green breaths are good for improving vision and for overcoming bad habits. It is soothing and cooling to most systems, but it should not be used for cancerous or tumorous conditions.

Blue Breath

Calming and soothing. Eases respiratory difficulty. Awakens artistic talents. Is generally healing for all children. Children with respiratory problems can benefit greatly by being taught to perform blue breathing.

Dark Blue Breath

Accelerates healing and mending after surgery. Helps heal bones (especially a teal blue) when combined with a tinge of green. Helps to open intuition. It can have a strengthening effect upon the endocrine system.

Turquoise Breath

Eases respiratory conditions. Is good for arthritis. Can be combined with pink to assist in overcoming bad eating habits. It, along with the blue breath, should be taught to children who have asthmatic or respiratory problems.

Violet Breath

Beneficial to skeletal and nervous systems. Purifying to the body. Helps detoxify. Awakens spiritual attunement. The violet breath can help align the physical and mental aspects of the human energy system.

Purple Breath

Helpful in detoxifying the body. Helps overcome strong obsessions and negative feelings. Most effective when combined with white. It can be used to alleviate conditions of infection and flu temporarily.

As you work with controlling the breath and activating color energies through it, you can easily transfer the healing to another person. You can transmit color healing by breathing upon the individual:

1. Determine the color most appropriate for the condition.

2. Have the individual recline.

3. Locate the troubled area.

4. Gently lay a colored cloth swatch of the appropriate color upon the area.

5. Gently hold it in place and begin rhythmic breathing to increase your own energy flow.

6. See and feel yourself filling with the color vibration.

7. Lean forward, bringing your mouth close to the cloth swatch. As you exhale, breathe strongly upon it. See and feel your colored breath energy penetrating the body and restoring balance. The warmth of the breath serves as a catalyst to activate the color vibrations.

8. Continue this breathing for several minutes, or until you are aware of balance being restored. This method of breathing color into another is very effective in easing and alleviating

pain. It is quite effective for headaches, cramps, and nerve problems. This healing can also be effected by breathing the color into the appropriate chakra center.

COLOR TECHNIQUE 4   *Color Therapy for the Chakras*

The ancient masters taught their students to be ever watchful. This meant paying attention to the various emotions and attitudes they were exposed to or experienced throughout the day. As they did this, they could then determine which chakra(s) was most likely to be unbalanced. They would then take extra time at the end of the day to balance these centers. Thus the imbalance did not get a chance to accumulate, ultimately creating or aggravating an actual physical problem.

We can do the same thing using the guidelines given earlier on the chakras. Listed for each were the emotions and mental attitudes that can cause or reflect an imbalance within that particular center. As we determine through our own self-evaluation the chakra(s) most likely to have been adversely affected, we can then take measures to correct them. Color therapy is simple and effective in this process.

We can use colors upon ourselves to balance and strengthen the chakras on a daily basis. One way of accomplishing this is through color breathing. Another, somewhat more complicated way is through making colored slides and sitting in front of a slide projector while the color is projected upon us. Although some metaphysical stores do sell such slides, you would probably have to make them yourself, using blank slide frames purchased at a camera store and theater filters of various colors.

One of the easiest ways of accomplishing this is with simple colored swatches that can be purchased inexpensively at any fabric store. Most fabric stores sell small felt and other cloth squares for around twenty to twenty-five cents apiece. They can be found in all the colors of the rainbow, thus they can be used to balance the seven chakras. They are also found in other shades as well. Once you have purchased them, you have an inexpensive tool for quick daily chakra therapy and color healing.

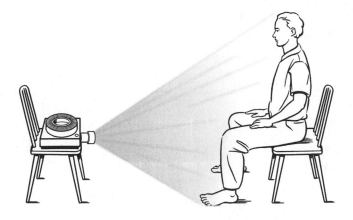

Using Colored Slides to Heal

1. Make sure you will be undisturbed for about fifteen to twenty minutes. It will rarely take any longer. Make sure the phone is off the hook, etc.

2. Lie down on your back on the floor or on your bed. Have seven cloth swatches with you (red, orange, yellow, green, blue, indigo, and violet), one for each of the seven major chakras.

3. Close your eyes and relax. Take several slow, deep breaths. As you begin to relax, look back over the day's events, in reverse order. Start with the moment you laid down and review the day backward until the moment you woke up. By looking over the day in reverse order, we concentrate more and we are less likely to overlook events and situations.

4. Note the major emotions and attitudes that you experienced or were exposed to in other people. What chakras were most likely to have been affected by them? Use the information on the chakras given earlier in this text to help you do this pin-pointing.

Chakra Color Therapy

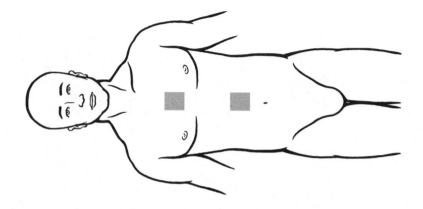

Begin by laying the colored cloth pieces upon those chakras you determined were most likely to be unbalanced.

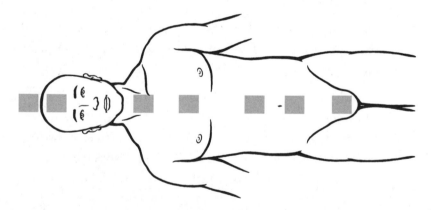

Next, lay the colored cloth swatches on each of the seven major chakras. Make sure you use the appropriate color for each center. Then just allow your body to absorb the energy for several minutes.

5. When you have completed this evaluation, take the color swatches for the chakra(s) you have identified, and lay them on the part of the body associated with the chakra.

6. As you lie there, with the color swatch upon your chakra point, visualize the color being absorbed and drawn through the chakra and into the body. Know that as you lie there, the chakra is being balanced, along with all organs and systems of the body associated with it. Take several deep breaths, focusing on drawing the color through the swatch into the chakra and restoring balance. Continue this for three to five minutes, or until you feel it is balanced.

7. Now repeat this with any other chakra you have determined may be out of balance.

8. Now place all seven color swatches upon the chakra points of the body. Breathe deeply and simply allow your body to absorb the rainbow energies. Know that as you lie there, each chakra is being strengthened, balanced, and harmonized with the others. Know that your entire energy system is strengthening. Feel yourself coming into complete balance. Know that all of the physiological aspects of your body are being balanced and healed as you absorb these colors through your chakra centers. Leave the swatches on for five to ten minutes or until you feel yourself fully balanced, charged, and aligned.

part 4

VIBRATIONAL HEALING
THROUGH THE
SENSE OF SOUND

eight

THE PRINCIPLES
OF HEALING SOUND

Sacred sound, whether as prayer, music, song, incantation, or chant, is a vital force. Sound has always been considered a direct link between humanity and the divine. At some point, all of the ancient mystery schools taught their students the use of sound as a creative and healing force.

Sound is a major contributing factor to our present states of health and consciousness. The difference between the random sounds of daily life and the focused use of sacred sound is that the latter produces harmony rather than dissonance.

When we learn to produce and direct specific healing sounds through our energy centers (chakras) into the physical body, balance occurs. Our entire energy system is strengthened. We have greater health on all levels, and we can disrupt negative qualities and patterns as they arise within our physical and subtle bodies. It all begins with understanding eight basic principles of healing sound:

- The Principle of Resonance
- The Principle of Rhythm

- The Principle of Melody

- The Principle of Harmony

- The Principle of Pitch

- The Principle of Timbre

- The Principle of Accumulative and Detectable Effects

- The Principle of Sound as Energy

The Principle of Resonance

Resonance is the most important healing principle of sound and music. It designates the ability of a vibration to reach out through vibrational waves to set off a similar vibration in another body. It is through resonance that the sympathy and antipathy to other people and conditions in our life environment can be explained. It is also this principle that allows us in the physical to contact and attune to those entities and energies in the spiritual or more ethereal dimensions of life.

The principle of resonance is most easily demonstrated through the use of a tuning fork and piano. If we were to strike a tuning fork keyed to the tone of middle C and then raise the lid on the piano, softly feeling along the piano wires, we would feel the piano wire for middle C also vibrating. The tuning fork triggered a response in that which was of a similar frequency. Even easier is to sit at the piano and depress the sustain pedal. Sing a note loudly and hold the note for three to five seconds. Now listen. You should hear the piano. Your voice has triggered a response in the piano wires closely in tune with your voice.

Every cell in our body is a sound resonator. It has the capacity of responding to any sound outside of it. Every organ, in which cells of like vibration have gathered to form that organ, will respond as a group to particular sound vibrations. The various systems in the body will also respond to sound vibrations, as will emotional, mental, and spiritual states of consciousness. The human body is a bioelectrical system that can be altered, strengthened, and/or balanced through the use of sound. This occurs through resonance.

By learning to direct and control our voice, use certain musical instruments, or apply various tones and forms of music, we can stimulate an immense number of sympathetic vibrations within our body and mind. Where there is imbalance, we can use directed sound and the principle of resonance to bring that imbalance back within its normal operating parameters.

Sympathetic vibration or resonance occurs when two or more bodies have similar or identical vibrational frequencies, making them more compatible. There is an innate sympathy.[5] This is sometimes called *free resonance*. An important factor is the individual's willingness and readiness to respond to a particular frequency.

This tells us much about the relationships we form. It is also because of sympathetic resonance that group rapport is established and individuals respond to the energies of others. In groups that come together for a singular purpose, the purpose serves as the medium for establishing sympathetic resonance among the participants.

Forced resonance occurs when two energy systems have different frequencies, and the stronger is transmitted to the other by force. This has both positive and negative aspects. Many forms and manifestations of cult activity (manipulation and abuse of mind power) can come as a result of forced resonance. It is through forced resonance that such phenomena as peer pressure occurs. The combined force of the group overwhelms the energy of the single individual and forces it into resonance with that group.

If understood and used correctly, forced resonance can overcome imbalanced conditions in the body, and thus bring various organs

---

5 Remember that humans are a microcosm of the universe. This means we have all energies and vibrational frequencies to some degree within us. It means we have an inherent ability to resonate with any vibration within the universe. This can be on a physical or nonphysical level, involving tangible and intangible energies. Even vibrations not recognizably physical but still affecting us can be sensed and felt if the intuitive and physical perceptions are heightened.

and systems back into their normal parameters. Forced resonance can be used to restore homeostasis.

The Principle of Rhythm

Rhythm is the pulse of life, and it affects all physical conditions. The drum beat of the Native Americans represents the heartbeat of Mother Earth. Rhythm can be used to restore a normal, healthy pulse within a person. Being exposed to a regular, steady rhythm triggers a similar response within your own body's natural rhythms.

Steady, directed rhythms restore the body's natural rhythms when they are out of balance. Individuals with heart conditions benefit strongly from listening to Baroque music with its balancing rhythms. It soothes and heals the pulsations of the heart.

In healing practices, rhythm (through drums, rattles, bells, etc.) can energize the body. Rhythms, especially those created through percussion instruments, activate the base and spleen chakras. These are linked to the circulatory system and the basic life force. These are our centers of sexuality—the physical expression of our spiritual vitality. Rhythms stimulate physical energies. Drumming can be a means of increasing blood flow through the body. The rhythms can quicken or slow the heartbeat and all organs associated with it.

Drums have long been used for many physical and metaphysical purposes. Whether the Tibetan ritual drum *damaru*, the North African drum the *tar*, or the Celtic *bhoudran*, drums and rhythms have both healing and spiritual aspects. There are rhythms for every occasion, internal and external. Part of our spiritual quest in life is how we each can personally discover and express our own rhythms. This the shamans knew and taught. It was how they healed and how they traveled to both heaven and hell.

It is wonderful that drums are being rediscovered. Everyone can learn to tap out a rhythm on it. You don't have to be professional, but we each can find that rhythm which comforts or sounds good to us. If it sounds good to us, it is healing and enlightening. To know a drum, you must play it. This can be studied literally, or as a simple metaphor for a healthy existence.

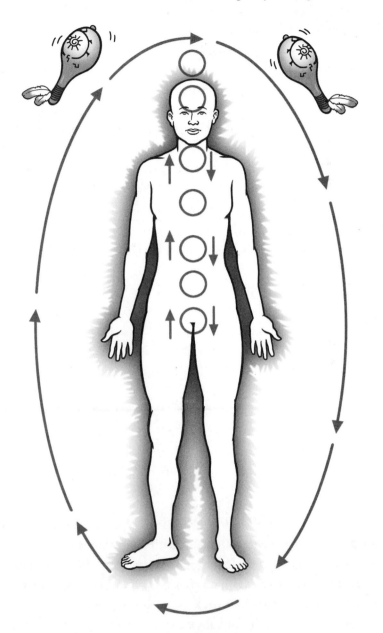

Shaking Up Negative Energy

The rattle is used in a variety of ways, depending upon the society and the illness. Regardless of the variation, there are some universal patterns to its use. The entire body is encircled. This loosens negative energy patterns that have lodged within the etheric body. Then the rattle is shaken up and down over the body to loosen the energy within through other methods by the practitioner.

Drum rhythms can trigger resonance within our own biological rhythms. An entrainment begins to occur, and our normal metabolic rhythms are altered to resonate with the rhythm of the drumming.

Research is beginning to reveal how different rhythms affect different physiological systems. I know of several people who are studying the heart and breathing rhythms of animals in hopes of duplicating them through drumming, so as to create resonance in their own bodies. When we consider that various animals never have problems with certain kinds of diseases, we may find in the drumming resonance a key to curing or alleviating what we once believed incurable.

Like its mate the drum, the rattle is also one of the oldest healing instruments. It is a cleansing instrument. It can be used to loosen rigid energy patterns that are establishing themselves within our auric field. This can be perceived like a static or snowy picture on the television screen. These patterns interfere with physical functions and normal metabolic rhythms.

The process of using a rattle is simple. It is shaken while encircling the body. The sounds of the rattle loosen the rigid energy debris and patterns. It is then shaken while moving it up and down the central meridians of the body (Governing and Conception). This loosens energy debris that has accumulated in these pathways and in the major chakras. Once the rigid energy debris is loosened, other healing methods can be employed to clear them out entirely.

The Principle of Melody

Melody cannot exist without relationship, and thus it helps us to see how everything is connected. One tone by itself does not create a melody, but as one tone is placed alongside other tones, melody is formed. Melodies—whether spoken, sung, or played upon a musical instrument—will soothe and alter emotional and mental stress that can be the cause of physical dis-ease.

Melody can be used to ease stress and relieve pain. Who has not seen a mother softly sing or hum to a crying child? (Often the mother rocks the child while doing so. This rocking activates the principle of rhythm and it helps soothe the child's metabolism.) The mother, by singing to the child, links her energies to the child (relationship), and the pain or distress is soothed and balanced. This is a gentle form of forced resonance. One of the most therapeutic activities we can perform regularly is to hum and sing simple melodies to ourselves. Doing so while on the way home from work restores balance and helps to cleanse us of any negative energy debris we have accumulated in the work environment.

Every melody is comprised of tones that affect us on many levels. The specific tones and their effects will be explored in the next chapter. It need only be light and simple, and you do not have to sing or hum it, or even be exposed to it for a great length of time. Anyone who has ever heard a child sung to sleep with a verse or two of "Brahms' Lullaby" understands this. Melody is one of the most ideal ways to relax and prevent physical illness.

The Principle of Harmony

Harmony affects our more subtle and spiritual energies. It is through harmony that the physical aspects of our energy can align with our more spiritual aspects. In harmony lies physical, emotional, mental, and spiritual aspects of sound. When working with harmony in healing, the simpler the harmony, the better.

A chord is two or more notes sounding simultaneously or in accordance with harmonics. Tones are blended together to create a unity of vibrations that a single tone cannot create. It stabilizes all systems in the body and brings them all into resonance with each other.

Working with harmony is the key to the alchemical process. It is the key to altering, transmuting, raising, lowering, and shifting our energies on all levels. It enables us to transmute major conditions of the body and alter states of consciousness. By finding the right combination of tones and rhythms and their harmonies, we can trigger a dynamic resonance that corrects and eliminates great imbalance.

Harmony reflects itself in all aspects of life. This is especially apparent in unfolding psychic abilities. As we work to develop one psychic gift (one tone), others awaken automatically and in harmony with the first. Those areas and systems of energy expression compatible with the first unfold and strengthen. This we can call spiritual harmonics.

The Principle of Pitch

Pitch must be considered in any of its forms when applying healing sounds. Pitch is the highness or lowness of a sound. The pitch is determined by the speed at which the sound waves vibrate. The faster the sound waves, the higher the pitch. Thus as we raise our physical and spiritual energy levels, we open to a higher degree of health.

Working with various pitch patterns can help us in shattering rigid energy patterns that are limiting our growth, awareness, and health. Specific pitches will affect specific chakra centers, and thus their corresponding organs and systems of the body. If a specific organ and its corresponding chakra are overactive or underactive, we can use a specifically pitched tone to bring it back into its normal range of operation.

The pitches for the chakras simply follow the musical scale. (Refer to the chart on the next page.) These pitches can be sung, played on a musical instrument, or experienced through listening to a piece of music written in the appropriate key, etc. Learning to sing or tone various pitches in our natural voice is a way of restoring our energies to their own natural level of homeostasis. Something as simple as singing and humming the musical scale can be stabilizing to our energy system and serve as a dose of preventative medicine. Some of these toning methods will be explored in the following chapter.

The Principle of Timbre

Timbre must also be considered in using healing sounds. The quality, the distinctive characteristics, and the influence of sound is called timbre or tone color. It is the distinguishing source of all sound. It

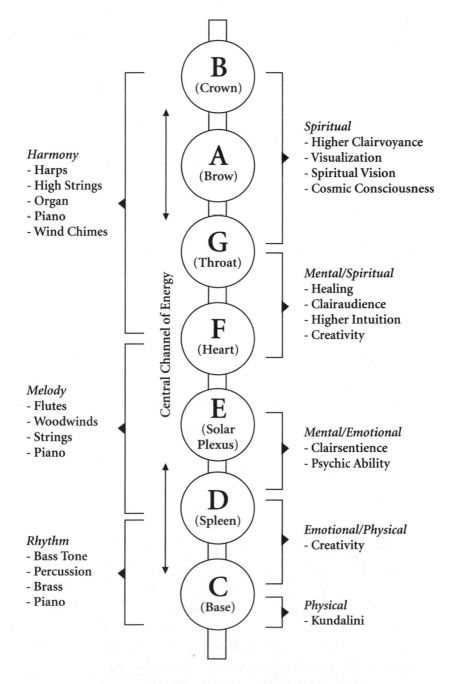

Metaphysical Principles of Healing Sound

helps us to identify one sound from another, one voice from another, one instrument from another. Every sound and sound instrument has its own distinguishable characteristic.

It is timbre, along with pitch, which gives us the greatest creative effects when applying healing sound. Timbre creates responses that are consonant or dissonant. Both terms relate to the energy perceptions of the body, mind, and spirit to outside stimuli and their effects. Different instruments, voices, etc., affect different chakras and systems in our body. (Again refer to the chart Metaphysical Principles of Healing Sound.)

When we respond with consonance to the timbre of various sounds (spoken or otherwise), we develop positive rapport. The cells in our body recognize what sounds are good for us and respond accordingly. The timbre of fingernails across a chalkboard is harsh and grating to the nervous system, while the timbre of a bamboo flute is soothing to the nervous system.

When we respond to sounds with dissonance, our energies are distinguishing those sounds that are not harmonious for us. Such sounds can be musical; they can be spoken as well—such as in the case of excessive criticism, whining, etc. Unless we pay attention to the signals that our bodies give us, we may allow detrimental sounds to impinge upon us unnecessarily.

Part of the application of healing sounds involves learning to control the timbre of the voice to create consonance or dissonance as is needed. Most of us do this naturally. If we wish to be left alone, we will assume a tone of voice that is harsher and more grating to others, pushing them away. If we wish to be friendly, we assume a softer, gentler, and lighter tone.

Through practice we can learn to effect physiological and spiritual changes in ourselves and in others through altering the timbre of our speech and by employing the timbre of various musical instruments to elicit desired effects. Some specific ways of adapting the voice timbre specifically for healing will be explored in the next chapter.

The Principle of Accumulative and Detectable Effects

The effects of sound are accumulative. The more we are exposed to beneficial sounds, the greater and more permanent effect they have upon our individual energies. The more we are exposed to detrimental sounds, the greater and more negative effects it has upon us on all levels.

Our bodies can discriminate between beneficial and detrimental sounds. These responses affect systems and functions of the body, as well as emotional, mental, and spiritual states. If someone criticizes us, don't we flinch and cringe? Our body responds to spoken sounds. Don't we catch our breath and cringe when we hear the sound of a crash? Our bodies respond to all sounds. Unfortunately, we do not pay attention to these responses. What holistic health and vibrational therapies should teach us is to be more perceptive. We know what sounds good to us. We are drawn to those who speak nicely of us, and we buy pieces of music that we enjoy hearing. We can detect what sounds are beneficial for us and which we need to avoid or cleanse ourselves of if we pay more conscious attention.

The Principle of Sound as Energy

Sound in any of its forms is a source of energy. As a source of energy, it can be used to interact with other energies. Sound—whether through music, voice, etc.—is an effective tool for altering electromagnetic fields and impulses of the individual and environment.

This means that if an imbalance has occurred within the body's normal electromagnetic parameters (whether it is a dysfunction of a specific organ or of a particular system), we can utilize sound in one of its forms or combination of forms to restore homeostasis, alleviate pain, and produce healing.

As an energy source, it can be used as a tool for a change of consciousness and to help discern the metaphysical cause of a physical problem. It facilitates concentration, relaxation, learning, creativity, and an increased awareness of psycho-spiritual states. It can interact and help alter brain wave patterns to facilitate this process.

General Methods for Employing Healing Sound Principles

There is no optimum method of employing the use of sounds and tones. It is good, though, to employ them for at least a minimum of fifteen minutes per session. You can use as many sessions as is necessary to alleviate a problem area, but no more than twice a day should be necessary. Remember that the effects are accumulative, so although you may not always see an immediate and tangible response, it will have a discernible effect, as you continue your efforts.

Experiment with different techniques. Music and sound are enjoyable. Take time to learn a little about music and the human body. The more we know, the more we can do.

You may employ these techniques as a general balm for all conditions; or if there is a specific problem, we can use them more directly to alter that condition. Begin by determining which chakra(s) is being affected. Determine which tone(s) would be beneficial for it. What colors and other vibrational remedies also would work with and enhance it? Do not be afraid to combine vibrational therapies. This will increase the effects tremendously.

1. Sing the musical scale to balance and align all of the chakras. If you are out of tune initially, continue until you are discernibly singing better. This is an audible clue that you have brought yourself into balance. Remember that we can discern when sounds are good for us and which are working.

2. Play a piece of classical music that has been written in the key for the chakra you wish to focus upon. (Do not worry that it may be written with a sharp or flat in the key, as it will still be close enough to be healing.) For example:

Base Chakra	middle C	Brahms' Symphony No.1 in C Minor
Spleen Chakra	D	Mahler's Symphony No.1 in D Major

Solar Plexus Chakra	E	Mozart's Symphony No. 39 in E-flat Major
Heart Chakra	F	Bach's Brandenburg Concertos in F Major
Throat Chakra	G	Bach's Brandenburg Concertos in G Major
Brow Chakra	A	Mendelssohn's String Quartet in A Major
Crown Chakra	B	Bach's Brandenburg Concerto in B-flat Major

3. Learn to play a musical instrument. It is never too late to learn to play an instrument. There are those that are relatively easy to acquire and learn. Recorders and bamboo flutes are but one example. You do not have to perform, but by learning to play the musical scale, you can use the tones to help heal and balance. Play the tones for the chakra that is imbalanced, repeat playing or hold the tone for several minutes. Follow up by playing the musical scale.

4. Inexpensive synthesizers can be easily purchased. These will enable you to use various timbres and pitches. You will be able to experiment to find which instrument's sounds have the greatest effect upon you. Most synthesizers today have percussion and extensive tone banks; thus they make wonderful healing tools.

5. Purchase an inexpensive pitch pipe at a local music store. Periodically play the pitches to restore balance. If you have been exposed to, or experienced, certain emotions and attitudes throughout the day, determine which chakra(s) is likely to be out of balance as we learned earlier in this book. Take several minutes at the end of the day and use that pitch pipe to balance. As you blow upon it, creating the sound, see and feel it being absorbed into the body.

6. Employ sounds and tones with etheric touch. If you are healing another, determine the chakra that is imbalanced. Hold
   your hands over it and perform rhythmic breathing. As you
   breath out, hum the tone or sound for that chakra as you project the energy through your hands. Try and feel the sound vibration moving through your body. This is especially effective
   when used with the toning technique described in the following chapter.

   You may also wish to see the tone as an actual color as you
   project it through etheric touch. Use the chart on page 155 to
   help you determine the sound and color correspondences appropriate for the chakra. The effects are intensified.

nine

TONING AND GROUP HEALING

We can employ musical rhythms, tones, instruments, and vocalizations to interact with the physiological activity of the body. We do not need extensive musical knowledge to do so. Everyone is musical. It is intrinsic to our nature. We have been surrounded and nourished by music since the moment of conception—from the sounds carried to us through the amniotic fluids during pregnancy, to the rhythmic beat of our own hearts. Music and rhythm are life itself.

Music is healing, and we should make it a conscious and active part of our health maintenance program. Even if we can't carry a tune or play a musical instrument, there are still simple ways of employing sacred sound in healing. If we can speak, we can heal with sound.

The voice has a tremendous ability to be an instrument for healing and nourishing. Throughout most of the world there has been a common belief in the healing capacity of the human voice. Shamans and holy men of primitive societies would utilize a spirit language to commune with higher intelligences to extract proper remedies. The Huichal Indians believe that the soul or consciousness emits a high frequency hissing or whistling noise. During times of illness, they believe the soul strays from the body. The Huichal shamans thus mimic this sound in order to help attract the soul back to the physical body to restore health.

161

Pythagoras recognized the considerable therapeutic power of human speech. He treated diseases through the reading of poetry. He taught students how a skillful, well-modulated voice, beautiful words, and their meter and rhythm could restore balance to body and soul.

Mantra yoga is a technique of human self-realization through the use of inner sounds (*nadas*) that are awakened through outer toning and chanting. In Tibetan beliefs, the most important musical instrument is the human voice, and the Tibetan shamans are trained in the use of outer vowel sound projection to create inner vibrations. They learn to use the head and chest as resonance chambers so that when the chanting stops, the sounds continue to echo within the mind and within the chambers of the body.

Each vowel sound, just as each musical tone, can open a particular part of the body when visualized and imagined during the in-breath and when spoken or toned internally. (Refer to the Table of Correspondences on the next page.) This inner sounding is the key to many metaphysical teachings concerning the healing sounds and mantras. Without the inner sounding before the outer, audible sounding, the effects are minimized.

The process of directed esoteric toning, beginning on page 164, involves both aspects, and it is easily learned and applied by anyone who can speak. Simply, as we inhale we focus our mind on the region of the body associated with the vowel sound, and we sound it silently. Then as we exhale, we vibrate or tone the sound outward and audibly.

This opening by the vowels can be understood if we realize that breath penetrates more or less deeply into the region concerned, according to our thoughts. The breath takes the energy of prana and, combined with the vowel tones, they open specific inner regions of the body or consciousness. (See the chart on page 165.)

With the aid of our thoughts and imagination, we can suffuse our whole body with sounds, restoring balance to all aspects of it. We can use the vowel sounds as an alternative to music in balancing and stimulating the chakras and their corresponding organs and systems.

Many people excuse themselves from the process of healing through sound, music, or voice by saying they can't play a musical instrument,

Table of Correspondences

Chakra	Tone	Vowel Sound	Mantram	Color	Attribute	Healing Property
Root	Middle C (Do)	ū (ooo)	Lam	Red	Vitality, Kundalini, Life force	Circulation, low blood pressure, colds, and shock
Spleen	D (Re)	ō (oh)	Vam	Orange	Creativity; Reserve-energy sexual	Muscles, reproduction, detoxifying, emotional balance, sexuality
Solar Plexus	E (Mi)	aw/ah	Ram	Yellow	Inspiration, intellect, wisdom, psychism	Digestion, laxative/constipative, headaches, adrenals
Heart	F (Fa)	ā (ay)	Yam	Green	Love/healing, balance, Akashic memory	Heart trouble, lungs, ulcers, hypertension, blood/circulation
Throat	G (Sol)	ĕ (eh) (ă/ŭh)	Ham	Blue	Clairaudience, cooling, relaxing	Throat, fevers, asthma, lungs, thyroid, antiseptic stimulation
Brow	A (La)	ĭ/ē (ih/ee)	Aum/Om	Indigo	Third eye, clairvoyance, spirituality	Purifier (blood), obsessions, coagulant, sinuses, headaches, stroke afflictions
Crown	B (Ti)	ē (ee)	Om	Violet	Christ Consciousness, inspiration	Soothing to nerves, stress, confusion, neurosis, insomnia, skeletal problems
*Soul Star (Transpersonal 8th chakra)	High C (above middle C)	——	Om	Purple or Magenta	That part of Soul linked to matter; link to our true spiritual essence	Building the Body of Light, key to burning away forms that hinder physical & spiritual health for discipleship

they can't sing, they can't go to a library to borrow music in the appropriate key, they can't afford an inexpensive pitch pipe, or any of a number of other reasons. But if they can speak, they can still heal themselves with sound.

Directed Esoteric Toning

Toning is the process of vibrating sounds and tones (musical and spoken) to assist the healing process. It is cleansing, harmonizing, and healing. It can be used to restore homeostasis to our entire energy system. It is also powerfully effective to use in conjunction with other vibrational therapies. It is one of the most powerful means of self-healing as we use our most creative musical instrument—the human voice.

Voice releases power. It releases it in the direction of our thoughts, thereby sending the energy to the appropriate area of the body. We can use the sounds for the entire chakra system, or we can focus on the toning for just a particular center or area of the body. An old axiom teaches "All energy follows thought." Where we put our thoughts, that is where energy will go. Where we focus our sounds and voice, the vibrations are carried there.

The purpose of toning is to restore the vibrational pattern of the body (physical and subtle), so that our spiritual essence can manifest more fully within the physical environment. Voice belongs to the body, but it is the instrument of the spiritual self. Being more than body, we need to learn to use it as a tool for higher consciousness and health.

1. Decide on the tone(s) to be used (the vowel sounds). Determine this by the problem area, the chakra associated with the problem area, or the emotions and attitudes experienced throughout the day.

2. Whether toning for yourself or performing it on someone else, be comfortable. Standing, sitting, or lying down positions can all be used; just make sure the spine is straight.

The Effects of Vowel Sounds

Vowel Glyph	Vowel Sounds	Chakras	Effects of Energy when Activated
A	ay (hay)	Heart	Chest, lungs, circulation, heart, mood (love, healing, balance, Akashic memory)
	ah (cat)	Throat	Throat, respiration, mouth, trachea, etc. (creative expression, clairaudience)
	aw (saw)	Solar Plexus	Stomach, digestion, left-brain, intestines (inspiration, clairsentience, psychism)
I	i (eye)	Medulla Oblongata	Balanced brain function, mental clarity (mind over emotions, "intelligence of heart")
	ih (bit)	Throat	Throat, respiration, mouth, trachea, etc. (creative expression, clairaudience)
E	ee (see)	Brow	Head cavity, sinuses, brain, pituitary gland (clairvoyance, third eye, spiritual vision)
		Crown	Skeletal system, pineal (Christ consciousness)
	eh	Throat	Throat, respiration, mouth, trachea, etc. (creative expression, clairaudience)
O	oh (note)	Spleen	Muscular system, reproduction, navel area (creativity, reserve energy, higher emotions)
	aw (cot)	Solar Plexus	Stomach, digestion, left-brain, intestines (inspiration, power, psychic sensitivity)
U	oo (boot)	Base	Genitals, pelvis, lower body, circulation (vitality, life force, kundalini)
	uh (but)	Throat	Throat, respiration, mouth, trachea, etc. (creative expression, clairaudience)

3. Focus on the center to which you will project the tone. In-hale slowly, sounding the tone silently within your own mind. Hold it briefly, and then exhale slowly, audibly toning the sound. Project it toward the appropriate area. If you are balancing yourself, focus your mind on that area or fold your hands over it as you tone.

4. Tone the sounds in the manner that is best for you. There is no specific length of time to hold and project the tone, nor is there any specific volume. Allow the voice to find its own volume and pitch. Try to keep the inner toning and the outer toning of equal length.

5. You may wish to sing the vowel sound in the appropriate note for the chakra. This can enhance the effects, but it is not necessary to effect changes.

6. Remember to inhale, toning silently, and then exhale, toning audibly. Silent, audible. In, out. Spiritual, physical. We are activating the dynamics of sacred sound.

7. Pay attention to your own voice as you tone. Your voice will act like a sonar instrument, providing you with input. If your voice cracks and fluctuates as you tone, repeat the toning of that sound until the voice smoothes out. This is your audible clue that balancing is occurring. At this point, continue the toning for several minutes.

8. You may wish to begin and end the toning session by toning the sounds for each chakra. In between, give extra toning to specific problem areas.

9. It is also a good practice to tone the vowel sounds for each chakra, starting from the bottom, at least once a day. It does not take long, and it will help you to maintain your own balance. Do several repetitions of the sound for one chakra before moving on to the next.

10. Experiment with various toning procedures. Employ the toning with etheric touch. Visualize the color of the chakra streaming forth as you tone the sound for the chakra. Combine your vibrational healing techniques. They all reinforce each other.

Breath is important to the process of directed esoteric toning. Breath refers to that quick intake or gasp of energy that carries an image or thought to the subconscious. All aspects of toning are related to breath. Breath is life. When we become aware of our breathing patterns, we have greater control over them. As we work with toning and become more balanced, our breathing becomes more fluid, healthy, and harmonious.

Experiment with the toning process. Take the primary vowel from your first name. Close your eyes and tone the sound slowly. Allow it to find its own volume and length of sound. Keep repeating, allowing it to find its own natural pitch. After a week of this you will find yourself toning this natural pitch. This helps develop greater resonance within your voice. Toning this sound ten to twelve times is balancing to the body and calming to the mind.

Work with all of the vowel sounds. Start with the base chakra and tone the sound five to ten times. Do this with each chakra. Use a pitch pipe and experiment on toning the vowel sound at different pitches.

Pay attention to areas in which you have difficulty with the tone or at those points where the voice breaks, cracks, or fluctuates. The voice acts like a sonar instrument. It provides feedback.

If the voice cracks and fluctuates, it indicates imbalance. Continue the toning until the voice smoothes out. This is an audible signal that balance has been restored. This kind of feedback is applicable when healing yourself or working on others.

Can you feel the sound in a particular part of the body? What is the effect? Is it comfortable? Agitating? Energizing? Relaxing? Determine the feeling as best you can. Do not be discouraged if you can't label it. Toning is a learning process as much as it is a healing process.

This toning process can be used to heal yourself and to increase self-awareness. As with all healing, relaxation is critical, but the unique aspect of sacred sound is that relaxation occurs as a natural part of the process. You cannot use healing sounds without it relieving stress.

Group Healing with Sacred Sound

The schools of wisdom had specific healing rooms and temples. Sound and music were a manifest part of their lives. The singing took the form of chanting, mantras, poetry, as well as the form we now call song. The toning process was also used. Groups of healers would tone or sing variations of sounds intimate to the individual. These could be prominent sounds within the individual's name or even the astrological chart.

A study of sacred geometry can amplify the healing effects of toning. Geometry affects the electromagnetic vibrations of the environment. Some geometric forms intensify, while others can soften the effects.

Individuals sometimes have difficulty believing that geometry affects us on any level. Look at your own home environment. In which room(s) do you spend the most time? The angles of that room may be affecting your own electromagnetic patterns, being more soothing to them. Look at the shape and angles of the rooms you spend the least amount of time in or that make you feel less comfortable.

Stories of Pythagoras abound about how he could translate musically the shape of the room, a building, or even a city. When we consider that music has a mathematics to us, especially in relating one note to another, or in converting sound to electrical signals, we begin to see many possibilities. It is not within the scope of this work to explore all of these avenues, but the bibliography will provide some sources for your own in-depth explorations.

How then can an individual with little musical background or knowledge of geometry work with the healing aspects? One of the most powerful means of healing through toning is in a group situation. Groups intensify the energies on an exponential level. Group healing is also one of the most effective for learning how to project and experience the effects. It allows many times more comfort in developing this ability.

Groups of healers can align themselves in various configurations around an individual to effect dynamic changes with sound. The use of geometric shapes around an individual while toning is very powerful. In the East, the use of geometric shapes is called *yantra* or geomancy. Yantras are essentially visual tools help in centering. When used for healing or worship purposes, the energy associated with the shape is invoked. When used in conjunction with toning, that energy becomes grounded into the physical to impact and help stimulate further the healing energies of the sounds. When the group members form a geometric shape about an individual, they create a vortex of energy within that shape. As they tone, the energy is set in motion.

Meditation and healing groups can have tremendous fun and experience wonderful effects by using them. It is a wonderful way of feeling and proving the effects of sacred sound to yourself. Each individual of the group can take turns being placed in the middle, while the other members form various geometric shapes around the individual. This also creates group harmony, and so toning is an effective process to do before any group ceremonial or ritual work.

Groups and circles are highly effective also for projecting long-distance healing tones to individuals. Depending upon the particular problem, the group must decide upon an appropriate geometric form and the tones that would be beneficial. Visualize the individual needing the healing as if he/she is in the middle of the group. If you have a picture of the individual, this can be placed in the center as well to further enhance the connection. As the group tones, they should visualize the energy going forth to touch the individual.

Symbolism of Geometric Shapes

A study of the symbolism of various geometric shapes will yield much fruit in using them for group toning and healing. The following are examples, and they by no means cover the spectrum of energies associated with the various shapes. Adapt the geometric shape to the group size, and don't be afraid to experiment.

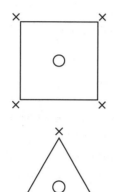 SQUARE—Forming a square about an individual while toning provides greater stability and equilibrium to the person's energy. It calms and settles when used with toning. It also amplifies and strengthens the life force of the base chakra.

TRIANGLE—The triangle will amplify and intensify the energies of the tones. It strongly affects the spleen chakra, and it can be used to heat up or cool down an individual's energy system when used with tones. It facilitates the toning to have an amplified cleansing effect.

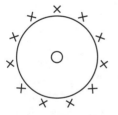 CIRCLE—The circle is the most natural and perfect shape in the world. It builds an energy vortex of totality and wholeness when used with toning. It harmonizes all systems of the body. It enhances the sounds so that they can create new life, health, and energy in the individual. The circle is the womb. It sets up a vortex that can link the divine with the human, the inner with the outer. It can be used effectively with toning, especially for any problems associated with the solar plexus chakra. It can be used when no other shape seems appropriate.

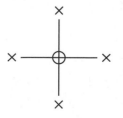 CROSS—The cross is a shape that sets up an energy that will balance the four elements of the body: fire, air, water, and earth. It strongly affects the heart chakra, especially when used with toning. It will help link and balance the four energies of the individual: physical, emotional,

mental, and spiritual. It creates a balanced polarity in the electro-magnetics of the individual. It balances the male and the female and it is stabilizing to all meridians when used with toning.

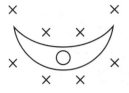

CRESCENT—The crescent is a shape that, when used with toning, will enhance healing of emotions and problems of expression. It is linked to the throat chakra and all energies of it. It can be used with toning to bring out the feminine energies of illumination, creative imagination, and intuition. It is a tremendous amplifier of toning effects, and it can be used almost universally for any toning procedure.

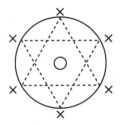

SIX-POINTED STAR—This figure, when used with toning, links the heart and the mind, the lower and the higher, the divine and the spiritual. It brings an alignment of the subtle energies with the physical. It strongly affects the brow and heart chakras. It can be used with toning to set up an energy that is strengthening and protecting. It helps stimulate inner solar fires that help in self-healing.

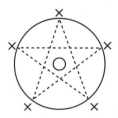

FIVE-POINTED STAR—This shape, when used with toning, is balancing and grounding. It is especially effective for the individual who is "spacey." It provides a concentrated force of energy. When used with sound and music, it draws those healing angels of strength and energy, especially those known as the Seraphim.

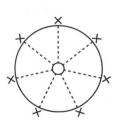

SEVEN-POINTED STAR—This shape, when used with toning, is extremely healing on all levels. Seven is the mystical number, and this figure assists in balancing all the chakras, subtle bodies, and physiological systems of the body. It creates a vortex that invokes the play of energies of the seven major planets more strongly.

It is soothing to the emotions, and it can be used universally to amplify the healing energies of children. (This shape is often called the Star of St. Bridgette, protector and healer of children.)

With each configuration, the person to be healed sits or lies in the middle. This is the strongest point of receptivity. The center is the nucleus of the circle. It is the focus of love, which is the healing energies of sound being poured forth by the other members of the group to the individual. It is only by being centered that we can re-establish health and balance.

Techniques for Applying Group Healing

1. Gather together a group of like-minded individuals. There does not need to be much more knowledge of the effects of sound than have already been discussed in this chapter and the previous one. The number of participants in the group is up to the group itself. The more members there are, the easier it will be to form certain geometric shapes. It also increases the power of the healing process, and will make it easier to still heal as a group during those weeks when certain members may be unable to participate.

2. Decide on regular times to meet. A weekly gathering can be beneficial. It is frequent enough to provide feedback from the previous week's efforts and it allows time between to experiment on one's own. It also allows for more working harmony among the group members. The stronger the group, the stronger the healing process.

3. Initially, you may not wish to try to heal anyone in particular. The first four to five sessions should involve creating group harmony and experimenting on each other so that each member of the group can experience the effects personally from the toning process.

4. Form a circle to establish a form of unity. Then review the directed esoteric toning process at the beginning of each session. Next, as a group, go through the vowel sounds for each chakra, using the directed esoteric toning process. Tone each vowel for each chakra at least three to four times. This general toning by the group will bring harmony, which is essential for the group energy to serve as a catalyst for healing. After several sessions, the group will begin to find its own levels of balance in regard to volume, pitch, and length of tone. You will begin to notice after several sessions that it is easier to find that group median.

5. Before working to heal others, it is best to experiment with all of the group members. The more experience the group members have in regard to the effects of tones, the more confident the group energy will be when projecting to others not of the group.

   One of the most beneficial exercises is to take turns being in the middle as the rest of the group tones you. Take a seated or prone position—whichever is more comfortable. Allow the group to form one of the geometric shapes around you and project at you the tones for each of the chakras. The individual in the middle should remain quiet with eyes closed, paying attention to what he/she feels.

   Then alternate. Each group member should have the opportunity to be toned while in the middle of the group. This should be done for each of the geometric shapes. Depending upon the size of the group, you may wish to do a different geometric shape each week until all have been tried.

6. After all have experienced the toning, take time to discuss the effects. Exchange notes on what you felt or experienced with others. Pay particular attention to similar kinds of experiences. Are there certain shapes that seemed to have a more dynamic effect than others for everyone in general? If

so, this may reflect a form that may be one of the most beneficial for the group energy.

7. Remind each other to pay attention to personal energy levels over the next few days—physically, emotionally, mentally, and spiritually. Discuss these observations the following week. It will help the group determine the extended, as well as the immediate, effects of the toning process.

8. Close each session with a group toning as well, back within a group circle. You may wish to reverse the process by toning from the crown chakra down to the root or base chakra center. This will help ground the group as they leave to go about their personal business.

9. Do not be afraid to experiment. Remember that in the early weeks, you are developing harmony and the ability to work together. An exchange of observations and personal experiences will be essential to help you understand how the toning can affect you and those you work to help heal. It will also help you to explain to those who come to you what they can or cannot expect to have happen.

10. As you begin to work on an individual, it is best to know how you will work in general as a group with that individual. One possibility is toning all of the chakras first while in a circle around the individual. Then move to the geometric form that is likely to be most effective for the individual's primary condition or health problem. Then tone as a group the sounds for the chakra most affected by the imbalance. At the end of the specific toning therapy, the group may wish to move back to a circle around the individual and tone the seven chakras once more to further strengthen the effects of the healing.

11. Don't be afraid to improvise. Each individual you work on will be different. Even though the group may have a set rou-

tine, this may have to be adjusted to fit the needs of the individual. Sometimes this is strictly an intuitive decision. It is a good idea to meet as a group thirty to forty-five minutes before the scheduled arrival of the individual to be healed if it is someone not from the group.

12. Alternate leadership. Each week, allow a different individual to lead the toning process. The leader should follow his or her intuition on how long to hold tones or whether to stay at a particular chakra center for lesser or greater amounts of time.

These are only guidelines. There will be little things that pop up in the formation and sustaining of group healing, but these are easily worked out. What works best for the group will work best in the healing process. You may wish to keep records and notes on those who come to the group for help and when. You may also want to do periodic follow-up to confirm the healing effects. This is important. Most people that you tone for will be happy to provide feedback. Oftentimes this feedback comes in the referral of others to you. As that begins to grow so does the group power, and you begin to become a true healing force in the lives of others and in the world.

part 5

VIBRATIONAL HEALING THROUGH THE SENSE OF TASTE

ten

THE POWER OF
FLOWER AND GEM ELIXIRS

F lower and gem elixirs are energy "medicines." They can be made and used by anyone. They do not interfere with any other form of traditional or nontraditional medicine, and they serve very dynamic functions in the entire holistic healing process:

- They can assist the individual in understanding the lessons of a particular illness or dis-ease that is being experienced.

- They can help restore physiological balance, as well as help balance emotional, mental, and spiritual states that have aggravated the condition.

- They can be used to help us open to new levels of awareness— and not just to those associated with health. This includes psychic, creative, and spiritual states of awareness and their integration within our physical life circumstances.

- They assist us in attuning to our environment. Because they are made from elements in nature, we begin to recognize through their use the intricate interplay of nature and humanity.

- They assist us in aligning and attuning to our more subtle energies and their impact upon our physical life.

- They assist us in developing a deva consciousness, an awareness of the archetypal patterns of energy that operate in and through nature. It is these patterns that enable each flower, plant, stone, and crystal to grow and form in its own unique manner, and yet do so in harmony with nature and humanity.

- Flower and gem elixirs are catalysts for transformation of emotional, mental and spiritual, thus repercussing upon the physical. (They do not act by way of a roundabout of the physical body, but rather they act upon the energy system at the root of and surrounding the physical body.)

In the 1930s, Dr. Edward Bach of London gave up a very lucrative practice to explore and develop remedies in the plant world that would restore vitality. The flowers were picked from various plants and trees and prepared into medicines that would create negative states of mind. He strove for simplicity, wanting to first identify the state of mind, mood, or personality, and then to pick an appropriate flower remedy for it.

The original thirty-eight remedies were discovered by trying them on himself. Dr. Bach was considered an extremely sensitive man who was so sensitive that if he placed the bloom of a flower upon his tongue, within a short time he would experience the exact state of mind that it would serve to heal. This reinforced his homeopathic training and its primary axiom of "Like cures like."

Unlike medicinal herbology, flower elixirs do not use the physical material of the plant. Instead the energy behind and pervading through the plant is extracted in a simple alchemical procedure. The flower remedies are truly "simples," as Dr. Bach referred to them. They stimulate no physical discomfort. They are only pure and beautiful elements of nature. The plants used in their making grow wild and free and most are accessible to anyone willing to search them out.

The 38 Bach Flower Remedies*

Agrimony—for inner torture behind a facade; awakens inner peace.

Aspen—for anxiety/apprehension; awakens openness to new experiences.

Beech—for criticalness; awakens acceptance and tolerance.

Centaury—for weakness of will; awakens inner strength.

Cerato—for lack of confidence; awakens trust in inner guidance.

Cherry Plum—for fear of collapse or shock; awakens courage under stress.

Chestnut Bud—for repeating same mistakes; awakens awareness of life's lessons.

Chicory—for possessiveness and martyr syndromes; awakens appropriate giving and receiving.

Clematis—for dreaminess and lack of attention; awakens a grounding and practical inspiration.

Crab Apple—for feelings of uncleanliness or shame; awakens harmony and an inner cleansing.

Elm—for feelings of inadequacy; awakens self-confidence.

Gentian—for discouragement and self-doubt; awakens perseverance and confidence.

Gorse—for despair and hopelessness; awakens faith and hope.

Heather—for self-absorption and failure to listen; awakens caring for others and ability to listen.

Holly—for jealousy, hate, and revenge; awakens compassion.

Honeysuckle—for dwelling in the past; awakens letting go of past.

Hornbeam—for lacking of strength to handle daily activities; awakens confidence of energy and ability.

Impatiens—for impatience and irritability; awakens patience and understanding.

Continued on next page

---

* Adapted and reprinted by permission of Ellon Bach, Inc. The material has been reported in the Bach remedies literature and should never be construed as a claim of efficacy. For further information, consult the references in the bibliography.

The 38 Bach Flower Remedies (*continued*)

Larch—for lack of self-confidence and inferiority; awakens confidence and creative expression.

Mimulus—for fears and shyness; awakens courage and confidence.

Mustard—for bloom and depression; awakens joy and peace of mind.

Oak—for despair and despondency; awakens brave perseverance and strength.

Olive—for mental/physical exhaustion; awakens renewed vitality.

Pine—for guilt and blame; awakens positive self-acceptance.

Red Chestnut—for excessive fear and anxiety; awakens calm detachment.

Rock Rose—for terror and panic; awakens courage to transcend self.

Rock Water—for inflexibility and self-denial; awakens flexibility, spontaneity, and self-nurturance.

Scleranthus—for uncertainty and indecision; awakens stable decisiveness.

Star of Bethlehem—for all shocks and trauma; awakens healing of trauma.

Sweet Chestnut—for despair and the last of endurance; awakens faith in darkest of times.

Vervain—for fanatical straining and overenthusiastic; awakens relaxation and moderation.

Vine—for domineering and inflexibility; awakens sensitive leadership and respect.

Walnut—for transition and change and over-sensitivity; awakens objectivity and freedom of perspectives.

Water Violet—for excessive pride and superiority; awakens humility and service.

White Chestnut—for unwanted thoughts and worry; awakens quietness and clarity of mind.

Wild Oat—for dissatisfaction in achievement; awakens clarity of life direction.

Wild Rose—for apathy and resignation; awakens enthusiasm for life.

Willow—for resentment and bitterness; awakens acceptance of responsibility and releasing of blame.

Ideally they are made from plants grown in natural conditions without chemicals.

Flower and gem elixirs are absolutely benign. They are not harmful or conflicting when taken with other medications. They cannot produce an unpleasant reaction under any circumstance. I have encountered individuals who complained of side effects, the most common being, "I can't handle the energy." In these cases, the individual is encouraged to examine his/her motivation for being ill and whether or not there is a true desire to get well. Remember, every illness and our response to it can teach us something about ourselves. The worst they can do is nothing. The best is they heal and enlighten.

There are as many uses for flower and gem elixirs as there are flowers and gems. Every flower has its own personality. Each flower and gem has its own vibrational frequency, its own life energy pattern. They each have their own unique function and effect upon the individual. A study of the flowers and gems, their colors, shapes, etc. can assist you in determining its energy pattern.

It is this energy pattern that is infused into a liquid. The liquid is then used to alter, transmute, or create new vibrational patterns for the individual—ones that will assist the individual in achieving particular functions and purposes.

However taken, the flower and gem elixirs are benign, although the course they take in healing an individual is not always predictable. Many experience immediate effects, with tension being relieved. Others find themselves able to confront aspects of the personality that helped the condition to manifest.

Some may not see the effects for up to seven days. Regardless of individual response, self-examination and even counseling are of tremendous help in working with flower and gem elixirs.

It is important to recognize the link between the psychological make-up and the physiological responses of the body for good or bad. The flower and gem elixirs assist us with this. Healing is not just removing physical discomfort or suffering, but it is also the coming to terms with the significance of the illness. The remedies stimulate opportunities for this self-encountering. If we want to return to true health, we must expect to change. Unfortunately, many of us are resistant to change. The elixirs open the consciousness to the higher self, bypassing personality resistances and blockages, to initiate the holistic healing process.

Beginning below are lists of other flower and gem elixirs. This is by no means complete, as there are hundreds of flower remedies available, and elixirs can also be made for every crystal and gem. Their descriptions, effects, and qualities are skeletal at best, but they will give you a starting point. In the bibliography are several works that provide in-depth information on individual flower and gem elixirs.

Read and study as much about flowers and gems as possible, as the information will provide much insight into the qualities of their elixirs. There are many commercial sources for flower and gem elixirs available, but it is beneficial to make your own—at least once. This helps you to attune to the alchemical processes of nature and its applications to your own natural energies. In the next chapter are specific directions for preparing and using your flower and gem elixirs.

Examples of Other Flower Remedies and Their Effects*

Angelica—opens one to the ministrations of the spiritual realms and angelic influences.

Blackberry—for manifesting creative inspiration and for opening to new levels of consciousness.

Calendula—awakens the healing power of words.

California Poppy—for higher intuition; assists in connecting with the nature kingdom and in seeing the aura.

Chaparral—helps one to experience deeper levels of psychic awareness and perception through dreams; helps in detoxifying the system.

Indian Paintbrush—stimulates artistic and creative expression.

---

* Adapted and summarized with permission from the Flower Essence Society, a Division of Earth-Spirit, Inc., P.O. Box 459, Nevada City, CA 95959.

Examples of Other Flower Remedies and Their Effects (*continued*)

Iris—stimulates creative imagination and inspiration; awakens artistic abilities.

Lavender—soothing to nerves and to over-sensitivity to psychic and spiritual experiences.

Lotus—for inspiration, intuition, healing; amplifies the effects of other essences.

Mugwort—awakens greater awareness of spiritual influence and understanding of dreams; assists in making you more conscious of your psychic energies.

Rose—awakens love and inspiration; helps attune to the angelic hierarchies and the divine feminine.

Rosemary—assists in controlled out-of-body experiences; stimulates mental faculties.

Sage—assists in awakening to inner world experiences; slows aging process; understanding life experiences.

Saint John's Wort—opens one to divine guidance; activates ability for lucid dreaming; increases psychic energies; assists in out-of-body experiences.

Shasta Daisy—spiritualizes the intellect; assists in seeing the entire picture.

Star Tulip—makes one more receptive to spiritual realms and astrological influences; awakens feminine aspects of imagination and intuition.

Sunflower—balances the ego and awakens the inner light of divine inspiration; assists in realizing capabilities of the soul.

Violet—attunement to the fairy realms; for awakening warmth and greater spirituality.

Wild Rose—for overcoming apathy and for integrating the spiritual in the physical; tonic for longstanding illness.

Yarrow—for psychic protection and oversensitivity; strengthens the aura; gives emotional clarity; eases stress.

Examples of Gem Elixirs and Uses

In recent years crystals, stones, and gems have become quite popular in regard to healing and higher consciousness. They are symbols and sources of specific energy patterns. A study of the basic properties and energy patterns of crystals and stones will provide insight into the elixirs made from them. It is this same energy pattern that is transferred to the liquid.

Base Chakra

SMOKY QUARTZ

This gem elixir will stimulate, balance, and purify the base chakra. It channels energy of the crown down to it so that it can be expressed more practically in the physical life of the individual.

It also grounds the expression of love. An elixir made from smoky quartz is strengthening to the entire auric field and helps to keep it clean of energy debris accumulated through contact with other people and environments.

Spleen Chakra

CARNELIAN (AND MOST ORANGE STONES)

An elixir made from carnelian and other orange stones help to awaken creative and artistic energies so they can be used by all aspects of his/her being. It helps us awaken our innate ability to manifest things. When used in meditation, it helps focus us on our goals and intentions, activating the magnetic polarities so we are more able to draw things to us. It can be used in health to alleviate anything associated with the spleen chakra, and it can also be used to tap into past-life records or information about a present illness that has its origin in a past life.

Solar Plexus Chakra

CITRINE

Citrine elixir helps to balance the rational mind and to open a bridge between it and the higher mental and intuitional levels of consciousness. It affects everything physiologically that the solar plexus affects, especially the digestive system. It awakens a greater sense of peace, relieving tensions. Like carnelian, it also activates the magnetic polarities of the body, and is good for those meridians that are yin. Citrine elixir can help us in clearly seeing higher goals, better health, and the best ways of manifesting them.

Heart Chakra

ROSE QUARTZ

Rose quartz elixir is a strong but gentle healing tonic. It helps in easing anger and in releasing negative emotions within the heart that are creating physical health problems. It can awaken a greater sense of inner peace and self-fulfillment. It is also effective for inner wounds revolving around past giving and receiving of love. It can be used for emotional release and for clearing our forgotten memories and energies that are blocking growth. It is good for all physical manifestations of emotional problems.

MALACHITE (ALL GREEN STONES IN GENERAL)

A gem elixir made from malachite awakens creativity and the energy and ability for change. It helps bring out true aspects and can be used in meditation to focus in on single problems. It should not be used in any physical condition that is tumorous or cancerous, as it can stimulate growth. It is good for strengthening the thymus and the immune system. It strengthens and stimulates the aura so that it triggers new opportunities for growth and balance.

Throat Chakra

TURQUOISE

Turquoise gem elixir balances emotional and creative expressions. It eases all imbalances associated with the throat chakra. It is especially effective in respiratory conditions. It heightens sensitivity, and it can be used as an aid to stimulate creativity and clairaudience. It protects those who work and live in negative environments, and it can assist the individual who is tied emotionally to other people's problems. It promotes healing on all levels.

Brow Chakra

SODALITE

Sodalite is the densest and the most grounded of the dark blue-stones. When used to make an elixir, it elicits deep thought and a clearing of the mind so that it can function properly. This elixir assists the individual in seeing which habits are helping to manifest the physical problem. It helps us to respond intelligently to all situations, and it helps us to reach logical conclusions about our health and other issues.

LAPIS LAZULI

An elixir made from this stone is very cleansing to the mind and the auric field. It can be used to break down subconscious blockages to deeper levels of consciousness and greater health. It can assist us in developing telepathy and in seeing what we need to do physically to clear a spiritual path for ourselves. It has a positive effect upon all conditions associated with the brow chakra.

FLUORITE

Fluorite is also an excellent elixir for the brow chakra and all conditions associated with it. It is multidimensional in its uses. It awakens in the aura a stronger energy pattern so that new opportunities can be discovered. It can help us in understanding the metaphysical causes of our physical problems. It is balancing to the polarities of the body, and thus can be used effectively with meridian work to balance the yin and yang. It is also balancing to the hemispheres of the brain and the nerve synapses connecting them.

Blue fluorite stimulates mental calmness. The purple fluorite as an elixir awakens our devotional aspects so that physical communion with the divine is easier. The yellow fluorite elixir helps us to understand our life experiences and their repercussions upon our health. The white fluorite elixir is purifying on all levels, and it assists us in uniting our own creative energies with those of the universe so that healing can occur more easily.

Crown Chakra

AMETHYST

Amethyst stones make excellent gem elixirs. They are cleansing and purifying on all levels. In many ways they are like blood purifiers. It can be used universally with all illnesses and diseases.

It awakens understanding and intuition when used in meditation—especially of health problems. It also awakens a greater sense of humility. It can also be used to overcome fears, and it can help open you to conscious astral projections.

Other Important Gem Elixirs

CLEAR QUARTZ

This elixir will augment the effects of all other flower and gem elixirs. It is effective in balancing and energizing all of the chakra centers. It is a good overall tonic. It awakens greater spiritual insight and helps us to express it within the physical. It balances and strengthens the aura. It is one of the easiest and most powerful of those elixirs made with crystal bowls.

MOONSTONE

An elixir made from moonstone can be beneficial to almost everyone upon the planet. It awakens and balances the feminine energies; and, since this is a feminine planet, it is essential to all life. It eases emotions, and it can help us move from lower emotional expressions to higher aspirations. This elixir also balances us as we cross new thresholds in our psychic and spiritual growth. For women, it is beneficial to easing the menstrual cycle and balancing all of the female hormones and organs. For men, it assists in recognition and expression of the feminine energies. It brings peace of mind.

Sources for Commercial Flower and Gem Remedies

The Dr. Bach Centre
Mt. Vernon, Sotwell
Wallingford, Oxon, OX10 OPZ
England

The Ellon Company (for Bach flower remedies)
P.O. Box 320
Woodmere, NY 11598

The Flower Essence Society
P.O. Box 459
Nevada City, CA 95959
(916) 265-9163

eleven

PREPARING AND USING HEALING ELIXIRS

F lower and gem elixirs are prepared by placing the flowers or crystals in a bowl of water (preferably a quartz crystal bowl) in full sunlight for several hours. They can also be made by lightly boiling the flowers and gems as well. Both methods will be elaborated upon in greater detail later within this chapter. This process extracts the life essence or energy matrix of the flowers and gems to form a potentized elixir. This is known as the *mother elixir*. To this elixir is added brandy or alcohol as a preservative.

From the mother elixir will come stock bottles. Two drops from the mother elixir are added to a one-ounce dropper bottle of good water (nonchemically treated). To this add a teaspoon of brandy as a preservative. From these stock bottles will come individual dosage bottles. The dosage bottles are also one ounce in size. Two drops of the elixir are taken from the stock bottle and placed in the dosage bottle. To this is added water and brandy. The flower and gem essences actually become potentized in this dilution method, much in the same manner as homeopathic medicines.[6]

Once the dosage bottle is made up, the individual can either take the elixir straight from the bottle or add drops to a glass of drinking water. Four to seven drops at a time are all that is needed, usually four times a day or as needed.

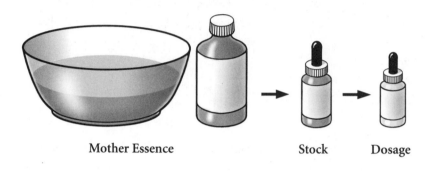

Mother Essence   Stock   Dosage

---

6 Dr. Ernst Lehrs, in the book *Man or Matter* (Faber and Faber), gave a description of the potentizing process as applied to homeopathy. "The method of diluting or potentizing, is as follows: a given volume of the material to be diluted in nine times its volume of distilled water. The degree of dilution thus arrived at is 1=10, usually symbolized as 1x. A 10th part of this solution is again mixed with nine times its bulk in water. The degree of dilution is now 1:100 or 2x. This process is continued as far as it is necessary.

"We can carry the dilution as far as we please without destroying the capacity of the substance to produce a physiological effect. On the contrary, as soon as its original capacity is reduced to a minimum by dilution, further dilution gives it the power to cause even stronger reactions, of a different and usually opposite kind. The second capacity rises through stages to a variable maximum as dilution proceeds.

"What this potentizing process shows is that, by repeated expansion in space, a substance can be carried beyond ponderable conditions of matter into pure functional effect. The potentisation of physical substances thus gains a significance far wider than that of medical use."

It is for this reason that the primary principle of homeopathy is "Like cures like." Disease symptoms are treated with highly diluted substances that produce similar symptoms if ingested in normal quantities. In the potentising process, the substance moves from cause to effect. The symbol of infinity reflects this process. As a

Often those who take energy "medicine" such as flower and gem elixirs must change their old ideas about medication. More is not better when it comes to these elixirs. Taking them upon rising, when going to sleep, and occasionally in between is all that is necessary. Also with flower and gem elixirs, increasing the frequency of dosages is more effective than increasing the amount of dosage. More frequent dosages are recommended for acute conditions and for accelerating the transformation process. Remember that we each have our own energy system, and thus there will be some experimentation to find what is best for you.

Making Flower and Gem Elixirs

The steps to making your own flower and gem elixirs are simple.

1. If you have access to a quartz crystal bowl, use it to make your flower and gem elixirs. A regular clear glass bowl can be used, but because of the lead in it, much of the light spectrum will be blocked and the infusing of the liquid with the energy matrix of the flower or gemstone will take longer and be weaker.

   Quartz crystal bowls are being sold in many metaphysical stores around the country as a dynamic tool for sound healing and higher consciousness. They are dynamically effective for creating powerful flower and gem elixirs.

---

substance to dilute and potentate, the inverse occurs. The cure or effect is elicited because the primal core of the energy is released. We are brought into touch with an archetypal pattern of energy that the body can respond to harmoniously.

Causes   Dilution (Potentizing)   Effects

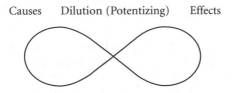

2. Clean the bowl you are to be using. A mild soap and water is effective.

3. Take time to meditate and attune to nature. Sitting and meditating outside, near the area of the flowers you will be using or outside with the stones and gems you will be using, is effective for establishing resonance with the remedy-making process.

4. If you intend to make gem elixirs, it is better to use stones in their raw and uncut form. If you do not have any in this form, do not be upset, just make sure that the stones and gems are cleansed thoroughly of any previous programming. Set them in sea salt, outdoors, for twenty-four to forty-eight hours before you are to make the elixir. This will serve to erase any programming and also charge them so they will more effectively imprint their energy pattern upon the liquid.

5. For the flowers, make sure you pick them in their full maturity, and do so early in the morning. The early sun is more vitalizing. Usually past noon the ultraviolet rays become more intense, and the basic prana of the air is diminished.

6. Have on hand appropriate water to use. Crystal spring water that is not chemically treated is most effective for flower elixirs. Distilled water is most effective for making gem elixirs.

7. Set the bowl in full sunlight. Make sure it is a day in which there are no clouds. Add approximately ten ounces of water to the bowl. If it is a quartz crystal bowl, chime it softly. I recommend twelve times to represent the movement of the sun through the zodiac. Remember that the more significance that we can add to the process, the more empowered the elixirs become. Chiming the bowl also serves to cleanse the water of any outstanding pollutants or thought contaminates.

8. Pick the flower blossoms and float them immediately upon the surface of the water. (Some people recommend that you handle the flowers with a leaf or stem, rather than your hands, and to avoid touching the water.) Float the flowers until the surface of the water is covered, making sure each blossom is touching the water. Place the bowl in the sun where the shadows will be unable to touch it for several hours.

9. After at least three hours—or until the flowers begin to fade—carefully remove the blossoms from the water. Use stems from the flowers or long crystal points to pick the blossoms out. I recommend the blossoms be laid around the shrubs and plants within the yard as a sign of reverence and as a blessing of the return to nature.

   For the gem elixirs, you may wish to leave the stones and gems in the sun a little longer. Some people recommend using brandy in the bowl with the stones, believing it to draw more energy from them than distilled water. Either way is effective. Using the brandy does help in purifying the stones. With raw cut stones, it is easy for dirt to become wedged in crevices in the stone itself, and using the brandy helps prevent contamination.

10. Ring the bowl again if you have a quartz crystal bowl. (Be careful of chiming it when stones are in the bottom, as it may cause a discordant vibration that can crack the bowl.) Then using a clean funnel, empty the contents into a dark brown bottle. You may also wish to strain it through cotton muslin. The brown bottles help preserve the life and energy of the elixir more than the clear.

11. Add brandy (approximately one fourth to one half of the amount of the elixir). This is your mother elixir. From it you will be able to make stock and dosage bottles.

12. On days that are less sunny or in poor weather, a boiling method can also be used to create the elixirs. In this procedure, the flowers are picked on as sunny a morning as possible. Fill a clean pot with the blossoms, and then add enough water to cover them.

13. Bring the water to a quick light boil, simmering for about a half an hour, with the pot uncovered. Then set it outside to cool. When the pot has cooled, cover it with a piece of cotton muslin and pour the liquid into a clean bowl. The cotton filters out sediment that occurs during the boiling. You may wish to pour from one pot to another several times, using the cotton to filter all sediment before pouring it into the bowl.

14. If it is a crystal bowl, play it for three to five minutes, and then set it outside for about an hour regardless of the amount of sunlight. If it is not a quartz crystal bowl, simply set it outside for an hour. This will help rejuvenate the energy imprint that may have been lost or weakened during the boiling.

15. Repeat steps 10 and 11 to create your mother elixir.

As you work with this process, you will have ideas for variations. Follow them. Flower and gem elixirs help us to attune to our more intuitive and subtle energies. It is important to begin to act upon them. Your own personal attunement and variations will help to form a foundation for a more dynamic use and response to the healing elixirs you prepare. Combine with the other. Although the combination may be compatible, you will not be able to determine and properly utilize its effects.

Charging and Storing Your Healing Elixirs

1. Place the elixirs in brown bottles. They filter out extraneous light (particularly artificial light) that can leech the energy from the stored essence.

2. Before use, shake the bottle of elixir. This keeps the energy active, and it prevents it from becoming dormant when not in use. Periodically shaking the bottles is beneficial.

3. Use dropper bottles for stock and personal dosage. This reduces waste and enables your elixirs to last a much greater length of time. Most pharmaceutical outlets sell empty dropper bottles. The primary sources for commercial essences, as listed at the end of the last chapter, often sell empty bottles as well.

4. When taking your dosage from the bottle (four to seven drops under the tongue), be careful not to touch the tongue with the dropper. This can serve as a transfer of bacteria to your dosage bottle. Occasionally, it is good to hold your bottles up to the light. If there is anything floating in them, they are contaminated, and you should not use them.

5. The elixirs can be charged and strengthened periodically. One method of doing so is to set the elixir bottle on a pad at the bottom of a crystal bowl and play the bowl for several minutes. Another method is to place them under a pyramid to charge them periodically. You may also wish to place a tiny quartz crystal inside each bottle. Quartz crystal is a dynamic amplifier of energy.

6. The mother elixir and stock bottles should be charged and cleansed about every three months. This keeps their energy matrix active.

7. Make sure you clean your items after making an elixir and before making a different kind, otherwise traces of one will

combine with the other. Although the combination may be compatible, you will not be able to determine and properly utilize its effects.

Determining the Elixirs You Need

Determining the flower or gem elixir to use is fairly straightforward. If working on altering a behavior pattern or personal characteristic, self-observation and common sense are the keys. How do you respond to various situations and people within your life? What qualities and abilities do you wish to develop? Which chakras are most likely affected? Asking yourself such questions can assist you in determining the elixir or combination of elixirs most beneficial to you.

Ideally, self-determination of the elixirs is encouraged, as opposed to having another choose the elixir for you. Counseling sessions and flower/gem readings can be effective in giving you insight and perspective, but ultimately it is your responsibility. "Know thyself" was a precept of the ancient mystery school, and this is the precept behind the use of flower and gem elixirs. They demand greater self-observation and personal responsibility if they are to be as dynamic a tool of healing as possible. They teach the individual to get in touch with his/her inner levels. Self-determination of the elixirs needed forces you to articulate the changes needed and to affirm the qualities desired.

In essence there are predominantly two methods for determining the elixir(s) to use. The first is a rational approach and the second is more intuitive. A third could be the combination of the two. Under each of these, though, there are specific techniques that you can employ.

The rational approach is done through the self-observation and questioning already discussed. Look at the patterns of your life. What mistakes do you tend to repeat? How do you respond to certain situations? How do you react to the people in your life? What are your predominant moods (especially for several weeks prior to an actual illness)? Observe yourself. Assess your needs and challenges. Keep in mind though that the qualities of all the elixirs apply to all of us at some time in our life.

Remember that Dr. Edward Bach worked to demystify medicine and develop a system that could be understood and used by anyone seeking better health. Read through the various descriptions of elixirs in this book and in those listed and described in the works found in the bibliography. Make a list of those remedies that correspond most to your personality type or to the stresses and emotions you are going through. List all of those linked to qualities you wish to develop.

Having made your list, decide which are most urgent or immediate. If undecided, rate them on a scale of 1 to 10 (with 1 as the lowest priority and 8 to 10 as the highest). You do not have to limit yourself to a single remedy, as they can be combined. It is best though to limit the combinations to seven or fewer. This allows the remedies to work more effectively together.

The other methods of choosing fall under the category of the intuitional approach. This includes such methods as using meditation to determine the elixir needed. Applied kinesiology can be used. Some individuals use etheric touch in the form of running their hands through the aura of an individual or over the tops of elixir bottles to "feel" the magnetic attraction or repulsion. Of all of these, one of the easiest of the intuitional is the application of radiesthesia.

Radiesthesia is a method of dowsing or divining to determine the elixir. It involves using a tool to determine the radiation of the elixir and its compatibility with the individual. It can involve the use of the pendulum, willow branches, dowsing rods, etc. It is a process of divining, of connecting to our divine nature that knows what we need. For it to work, the mind must be kept objective, but it is a method that anyone can easily learn and develop to a high degree.

Making and Using a Pendulum

Of all the tools of radiesthesia, the pendulum is easiest. A pendulum is made by attaching a symmetrical object to the end of a thread or chain. It is then dangled over the object in question. It provides answers to our questions in accordance with its movement.

Steps to Using a Pendulum

1. Draw a circle on a piece of paper. Place horizontal and vertical lines through the circle. You may wish to draw an inner circle in which to place a witness (if you are divining for someone else) or a particular elixir that you wish to assess. Refer to the diagrams on the following pages. With a little ingenuity, you can turn this circle into a powerful assessment tool for yourself.

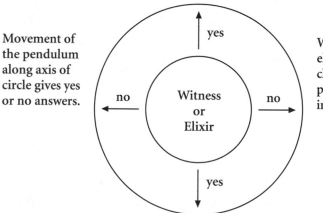

Movement of the pendulum along axis of circle gives yes or no answers.

Witness or elixir to be checked is placed in the inner circle.

yes

no   Witness or Elixir   no

yes

2. Decide what each direction or movement will mean. If the pendulum swings in the vertical direction, is it an affirmative answer? If it swings horizontally, is it a negative response? Whatever you decide the movements will mean, hold to that whenever you use the pendulum henceforth. You are laying the ground rules for your intuition to communicate to you through the symbology of the movement. Common movement assignments are:

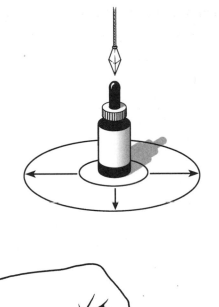

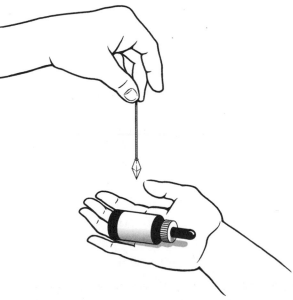

Using the Pendulum to Divine the Elixirs

Place elixir within the inner circle as in the top illustration, hold the pendulum over it, and ask your questions about its appropriateness to your condition. You may also hold the elixir in one hand while you divine its benefits with the pendulum in the other hand.

- Back and forth along the horizontal line = NO
- Back and forth along the vertical line = YES
- Clockwise circling = YES
- Counterclockwise circling = NO

3. Practice with the pendulum before using it on yourself and others to determine flower and gem elixirs. Set the circle flat upon a table. Rest your elbow on the table so that your hand is above the circle. Hold the pendulum thread between the thumb and first finger, with the weighted end dangling an inch or two above the heart of the circle. Ask yourself some yes and no questions that you know the answer to. Initially, move the pendulum so that it swings in the direction of the correct answer. At this point, you are simply sending messages to the more intuitive levels of your consciousness, letting it know how to communicate to you through the pendulum.

4. Next set the elixir in the inner circle. Hold the pendulum over it. Make sure it is not moving. Then simply ask appropriate questions: "Do I need this flower/gem elixir?" "Does _____ need this flower/gem elixir?" The movement and the strength of the movement will give you your answer. Remember that it is the intuitive level of the mind that is interacting with the energy of the elixir and causing the movement of the pendulum to respond accordingly.

   If you wish, you can also hold the elixir in one hand, while testing it with the pendulum with your other hand. You can also determine elixirs for someone at a long distance. Place a witness (something that represents the individual) in the inner circle, along with the elixir. Then ask questions. Remember these are guidelines to help you develop a quick attunement to your more intuitive levels.

5. You can also use the pendulum to provide guidelines for dosage and combinations that are beneficial. It all depends on the questions you ask. Be specific and phrase in a "Yes" or

"No" pattern: "Do these three elixirs work well together for me?" "Should I take these elixirs four times a day?" "Five?" etc.

Remember that the pendulum is a tool for communicating with the subconscious mind—the seat of our intuitive energies. The subconscious intuition communicates through the nervous system, giving signals that make the pendulum move.

The swinging of the pendulum is an ideo-motor response—an involuntary muscle reaction caused by the subconscious mind. Any muscular action creates electrical impulses, which are transferred in this case through the hand and into the pendulum, causing it to move in the appropriate manner.

Some Last Thoughts on the Flower and Gem Elixirs

Children respond strongly and effectively to vibrational remedies such as elixirs. Their energy systems on the whole are more magnetic, and thus they absorb the outside vibrations into their system easily.

The flower and gem elixirs are dynamic tools of preventative medicine with children. They can be used to strengthen and build the child's immune system and to keep the child balanced and attained to those more intuitive energies. With children, it is beneficial to lessen the number of essences within combinations as their systems respond so strongly to these elixirs.

The elixirs can also be used with the treatment of pets for illness and personality quirks. Simply adding the elixir to their food and to their water is the easiest method.

part 6

VIBRATIONAL HEALING
THROUGH THE
SENSE OF SMELL

twelve

THE WONDERS OF
INCENSE AND OILS

Oils and incense provide some of the most beautiful and effective means of raising or changing our own vibrational levels physically or otherwise. By learning to utilize the vibrational energy of fragrance, we can tap resources of energy and power and manifest greater health. The procedures for doing so are neither complicated nor esoteric.

We each have surrounding us an individual energy field, called the aura. By effecting changes within the auric field outside of the body, we can trigger responses internally. This sympathetic energy response can be used for a variety of manifestations, health or otherwise. Fragrance, like color, sound, and thought, is a vibrational force that we can easily learn. There are three principles of vibrational energy that are so easily demonstrated through the use of fragrances. The first we have already discussed. It is that all energy follows thought. Where we focus our thoughts, we focus energy of a particular frequency. If we then add another focus—one that is in harmony with our thoughts—the energy is strengthened and magnified, eliciting more dynamic results. Our focus of thoughts is more concentrated.

This triggers a second principle, sometimes called the law of correspondence. This law states, "As above, so below; as below, so above." What we do on one level affects us on all other levels. There is resonance between all things and all expressions of energy at some point. The vibrations that we focus with our thoughts and then magnify through other vibrational methods (i.e., color, sound, elixirs, fragrance, etc.) will seek out that which is of a similar vibration—whether it is outside of the body or of a pattern inside the body—and trigger a response.

Hidden within this second principle is the third, which is sometimes called the law of attraction—"Like attracts like." The body is a microcosm, and we can use a fragrance to impact upon the aura and thus attract inwardly those energy patterns that are needed. This can be used to strengthen a system, an organ, or any bodily function. It can also be used to open creativity and intuition, if we know what force to use to trigger the response. In the next chapter we will cover over thirty fragrances (aromatic forces) that can be used to stimulate mind and body for greater health.

Learning to use oils and incense can help us create an energy field around us that is strong and vibrant. We can use them to restore health and balance, and we can use them to awaken awareness of innate ability.

Every oil and incense will alter the vibrational rate of the environment and the individual according to its own unique properties. They most strongly affect the etheric, astral, and mental energy fields of the individual.

Oils and incenses have been used to counter the effects of dis-ease and illness, whether physical, emotional, mental, or spiritual. Some oils kill bacteria and organisms encountered within the air, on the walls, or in the human body. The aroma permeates the body primarily through the olfactory nerves, connecting into the brow chakra and the pituitary gland—the controlling gland of the endocrine system.

There is not always an immediate resonance between the fragrance and the individual, but by working on and using the aroma repeatedly, resonance can be established. This occurs because each fragrance has the ability to resonate with some aspect of our energy system, but it is usually our more physical energies that may tend to find the fragrance initially discordant and disruptive.

Incenses

Most of the early incenses were made from barks and dried herbs and plants. Each had its own unique characteristics. This book is not designed to go into all of these, but there are sources listed in the bibliography that can assist you in further explorations.

Incense is an excellent adjunct to any form of elevation of consciousness. There has been a long-held belief that specific angels tend to the various incenses. As the incense burns and the smoke rises, the thoughts and prayers of the individual rise also to be tended to by the angelic kingdom.

In healing work, the incense can be used to cleanse the auras, to open or stimulate meridian activity, and to invite spiritual assistance in the healing process. There are mainly two types of incense:

- ACTIVE—This incense has a commanding and stimulating effect. It is often used for invocation and materialization work in ritual and mediumship. It raises the energy levels and consciousness of the individual. Active incenses can be used for individuals who have health problems due to a slow or sluggish metabolism. It can be used to stimulate the yang meridians. Frankincense, sage, and incenses made from the mint family are examples.

- PASSIVE—This kind of incense is relaxing and soothing. It has the effect of opening the person. It stimulates the magnetic or yin qualities of a person. It helps the individual to go within himself or herself to find the source of the imbalance when used in healing meditations. They can calm and ease inflamed conditions and slow metabolic processes that are overactive.

Sandalwood, rose, and patchouli incense are examples of passive scents.

Some people feel that incense should be simply a part of the background in any meditation, ritual, or healing work, but there are others who use its attendant thoughtform as an integral part of the work itself. Incense actually has many uses:

- It can be used to mask or neutralize unpleasant smells. It was often heavily used in the past to ease the smells when the dead were being prepared to be buried. Confucius once said that while candles illumine men's hearts, incense perfumes bad smells.

- Pleasant aromatic odors are considered pleasing to various deities or divine forces.

- Incense is also a medium for prayer. As the smoke rises, it carries with it an individual's petition to the divine.

- Incense creates an atmosphere conducive to healing and resonating with a force to draw higher beings. Smudging, as done by the Native Americans and others involved in spiritual work, was done with incense. It was a way of cleaning the environment and the aura of the participants.

- Incense also has uses to treat the ill. It can cleanse the aura and effect changes in meridian processes within the body.

- Incense can be used to facilitate meditation and initiation into higher states of consciousness.

- Incense has also been used to receive revelation from spirits, to gain affection, to secure friendships, to succeed in business, and even to astral project. Incense can be used to enhance almost any activity humans are involved in.

The most common manner of using incense is in the form of joss sticks. Some cheap incense is still made with toxic elements, so as they burn, the toxins are also released. Most good incense manufacturers label their packets as being free of toxic substances and/or made from all-natural substances. You can also burn charcoal and use loose dried herbs, barks, and powders with it. The effects are not as long lasting as the joss sticks, but the fragrances are often more true and more aromatic.

Simply allow the incense to burn in the room where you are working. You may also brush or wash the smoke over you or parts of the body to effect more intimate changes. Some experimentation is necessary in employing incense in healing, but that makes it more enjoyable.

Essential Oils

Essential oils have been used throughout history for several purposes. The first is for their therapeutic use. They are dynamic aids in healing and in restoring bodily health. The second primary use is for the spiritual upliftment that they can bring to the individual. They alter the aura of the individual, affecting internal energy systems, and they affect the environment according to the quality and characteristic of the individual oil.

Oils have also been used in the preparation process when death is near. They were intended to aid the normal process of nature by freeing the body from lower influences, opening it to higher. The body (especially the chakra energy centers) was anointed in specific oils to seal the force centers so that after death, other entities were prevented from entering the body shell.

Most essential oils are made through a complex distilling process. They are very potent and intoxicating, and they comprise a strong facet of holistic medicine known as aromatherapy; the primary purpose of oils throughout history and even today is their ability to give relief to those suffering from various illnesses.

Essential oils are usually classified as being high-note or low-note fragrances. Low-note fragrances are heavy, thick, and often musky and earthier. Their ability to effect change is not as quick as high notes, but their effects do last longer. They are often well suited to hyperactive people.

High-note fragrances lean more to the light, sweet, and airy smells. The fragrance of high-note oils acts quickly upon a person, but they also dissipate and evaporate more quickly as well. Their effects are not sustained as long as low-note fragrances. When oils are used in combination, it is usually the first thing smelled, and they are better for sluggish individuals.

One way of working with essential oils is through combinations. Combine and blend low-note fragrances and high-note fragrances. It is pleasurable and it helps you to find the combination, the ideal fragrance, that has the most beneficial effect upon you.

How to Use Essential Oils

1. They are very potent, and thus you must be careful about sticking your nose next to the opening of the bottle and inhaling deeply. This will burn away the olfactory nerve. Instead, put a dab on a cotton ball and occasionally bring it to the nose. You may also uncap the bottle and with your hand, coax and wave the aroma up to you. Smelling several, one after the other, can diminish your sense of smell.

2. They can also be used like a perfume. You must be careful, though, as many essential oils are harsh and can burn and irritate the skin. It is best that they be diluted. Also, test a drop on the inside of the arm before you place any of the oil on more sensitive areas.

3. A drop (preferably diluted) can be massaged into a particular problem area.

4. A drop can be diluted in a small container of water, and this can be massaged into the meridian pathway that is most affected by the aroma.

5. Essential oils are very antibacterial. They can thus be used effectively in wash water for floors, walls, clothes, etc.

6. Taking a bath in an essential oil is not only healing but soothing as well. A half capful per tub of water is all that is needed. In this way, the fragrance is able to touch your entire body, and you take its aroma and energy with you when you get out.

7. Essential oils can also be used in vaporizers and potpourri pots to fill a room with a particular fragrance for an extended period.

8. You can also take a small bowl of water, place a drop or two of essential oil in it, and set it next to your bed. You are treating yourself to aromatherapy while you sleep.

9. There are expensive diffusers now out on the market that continually put the fragrance out into the air for extended periods of time. It only takes a drop or two of oil. Although expensive, they do use less oil than the other methods.

10. You can also place a drop or two on a light bulb. As the light bulb heats up, the fragrance is given off to fill a room with a particular aroma.

Using essential oils is a dynamic way to set a mood or a tone. Depending on the fragrance, you can stimulate lightheartedness, seriousness, joyfulness, or healing. One of the ways I have found them to be effective is in setting the energy for a healing. Usually if I am doing a session with someone—be it healing, counseling, etc.—I will use a fragrance in the room where I am working that is appropriate to the session. When the individual arrives, the energy of the fragrance immediately interacts with their aura, bringing it into a particular vibrational frequency. This makes my efforts easier.

Oils are dynamic tools, but they are enjoyable as well. As we work to mix and match and find the right combinations, we not only enjoy the wonderful benefits of the fragrances ourselves, but we develop greater confidence in ourselves because we are doing something physical to help ourselves.

A Simple Anointing Technique

When we give a blessing, a healing, or an anointing with oil, our state of mind and our sincerity is of great importance. When we anoint anyone, either when they are sick or to help them get rid of negative energies, we must first decide which oil(s) will be the most beneficial. Perform an analysis of the attitudes, emotions, or physical dis-ease and determine which chakra(s) is most likely to be affected. Then choose the oil(s) accordingly. The list in the next chapter will assist you with this. Then simply follow these steps.

1. Begin by preparing yourself. Do a progressive relaxation, and make sure you are balanced and centered.

2. Prior to the individual arriving, cleanse the environment. Either smudge with a strong, purifying incense, or by perfuming the environment through one of the methods listed earlier. Have fragrances and clean cotton balls available.

3. When the individual arrives, have him/her lie down, face up. Have them close their eyes and take several nice, long, easy, deep breaths. As they begin to relax, talk to them in a soft voice, explaining what you are going to do and with what fragrances. It is important to ease any anxiety before working on the individual.

4. Begin your own rhythmic breathing. See and feel yourself filling with a dynamic healing energy, an energy that you will transmit in the anointing to amplify its effects.

5. Hold the cotton between the thumb and the Saturn finger of the hand (the middle finger), and dab the oil onto the cotton. Using this cotton swab, anoint the area. This may be a specific area of the body or the chakra center of concern. There are several ways of performing the anointing, and you can simply decide which is right for the occasion or you may find that there is a way of anointing that is unique and more effective for you:

- You may anoint the area in small clockwise circles.
- You may trace the imbalanced meridian with the cotton swab.
- If it is a chakra center, you may draw the geometric shape for that chakra over that area of the body. Use the geometric shapes given in chapter 9 as a guideline.

6. Ideally, the body should be anointed directly, but depending on the occasion, the individual involved, decorum, etc., the anointing may have to be done through the clothing.

7. After anointing the specific problem area, you may wish to culminate the activity with an anointing of all seven chakra centers. You may also want to use this in conjunction with toning, color, and etheric touch. It is effective alone or in combinations.

thirteen

COMMON HEALING
FRAGRANCES AND THEIR USES

T he following are some of the most effective cleansing and healing fragrances. They can be found in the form of incense and
essential oils. The descriptions are not prescriptive. They simply reflect ways in which they have been applied in the past. They are
guidelines to beginning your own exploration of vibrational therapy
through the sense of smell.

APPLE BLOSSOM—This fragrance is soothing to the emotions. It
promotes happiness, an aura of success, and it enhances all aspects of healing. It is cleansing to the astral body and helps in discovering physical problems manifesting through inappropriate
love. In meditation it is useful in linking with the unicorn who,
myths tell us, lives under the apple tree.

BAY—This fragrance is very penetrating. It is good for lung conditions, and thus the Lung Meridian. It is healing and balancing to
the heart and throat chakras, and all conditions associated with
them. It is effective in treating colds. It is very antiseptic and
decongestive.

BAYBERRY—Bayberry is balancing to the spleen and heart chakras, and thus it eases emotions and illnesses resulting from unbalanced emotions. It helps align the astral and mental bodies with the physical, especially in times of great distress and turmoil. It is soothing to the entire auric field, and it eases fears about money and finances.

CARNATION—One of the most ancient and powerful healing fragrances, carnation was often used to anoint the heads of the sick to hasten recovery. It stimulates the entire metabolism and the energy flow throughout the entire body. It temporarily balances and removes blockages in all of the meridians. It is an excellent tonic fragrance, as it helps restore energy after exertion. It is strengthening to the aura so that we are less likely to be impacted upon from outside energies. It was worn during Elizabethan times to ensure avoiding untimely death upon the scaffold.

CHAMOMILE—Chamomile fragrance augments the entire nervous system. It is strengthening to the respiratory system, the endocrine system, and the Kidney Meridian. It helps release emotional tension that is the cause of physical problems. It is calming to the stomach and can be used effectively in anointing the Stomach Meridian. It is good for colic in children. It helps balance the polarities in the meridian flow. The fragrance has many of the herbal properties that relieve stress and aid digestion. It is protective to the energy field. It is also part of the ragweed family, and so those with allergies may want to be careful in its use.

CINNAMON—Cinnamon will magnify the effects of most fragrances and incenses. It can be mixed with sandalwood for deeper meditations. It enhances healing on all levels, especially the yang meridians of the body. It is a good fragrance to have if there is a need for psychic protection.

CITRONELLA—This is a protective oil, and it is strengthening to the auric field. It has a strong effect upon the throat chakra and all conditions related to it. It can be used to stimulate expression and communication, especially in those who are reluctant or hesitant to express feelings.

CLOVE—Clove was used in wash water in the mid-nineteenth century to help fight the tuberculosis bacilli. It is very antiseptic. It balances and evenly distributes spleen and heart energies. It's also good for memory, eyesight, and muscular and nervous tension. It was used for protection and exorcisms as well. Its fragrance is comforting to the bereaved.

EUCALYPTUS—A dynamic healing oil that should be a part of every household. It has a strong effect upon all of the yin meridians. Its penetrating quality is effective in treating conditions of the lungs, kidneys, liver, and nasal passages. It can be used for asthma, jaundice, and sinus disorders. It helps the eliminative system dispel toxins. It balances the heart chakra and stimulates the immune system. It is very effective in easing grief and hostility. It strengthens the meridians and augments the activities of other vibrational remedies. It eases disturbed sleep. A few drops in a bowl of water at night will ease nightmares, and balance and calm emotions.

FRANGIPANI—This fragrance strengthens the aura in a way that lets others see you as more confident. It helps open the throat chakra, and thus people are more likely to speak, confide secrets, etc. It temporarily balances the polarities of the meridians. It is excellent to use in meditation.

FRANKINCENSE—Frankincense is a sacred, ancient fragrance. It has often been used in anointing the sick and for cleansing the environment and aura. It is a purifier, and it can help shed light on obsessions and how best to break them. It can be used to induce a stronger vision of health, and it affects the crown chakra and all conditions associated with it.

GARDENIA—This fragrance strengthens the aura in such a manner that people are less likely to create strife in your life. It is one I recommend to healers, counselors, etc., as it helps prevent becoming emotionally tied into other peoples' problems. It is stabilizing to those who work with emotionally disturbed people. It helps repel negativity so that it does not get a chance to manifest in the physical body. It has a very high spiritual vibration, and it can also be used by individuals to connect with the nature spirits. It also enhances the development of telepathy.

HONEYSUCKLE—This fragrance is strengthening to the brow and crown chakras. It helps with problems of memory and it balances the hemispheres of the brain. It stimulates flexibility—bodily and emotionally and mentally. It also helps awaken psychic abilities.

HYACINTH—This fragrance is good for the Conception Meridian. It relieves grief and depression, and it will balance the spleen and base chakras and all conditions associated with them. It is also good for temporarily balancing the yin and yang meridians in the body. It can be used to ease insomnia, and it can help ease the pain of childbirth.

JASMINE—This fragrance was considered sacred in ancient Persia. It raises the self-esteem and it strongly affects the heart chakra and the Heart Meridian. It is good for nasal and lung conditions. It improves the sense of smell, so anyone who does extensive aromatherapy can benefit from it. It stimulates mental clarity and practicality, and also can facilitate the childbirth process. It eases times of great transformation.

LAVENDER—Lavender as an herb has always been considered magical, one that can provide protection, especially from cruel treatment by spouses. It is also a fragrance that every household should have because of its healing abilities. It is relaxing to the entire body, relieving it of stress. It is good for headaches, insomnia, pains, sprains, neuralgia, arthritis, toothaches, rheumatism, and depression. It activates the crown chakra and stimulates activity of the medulla oblongata, bringing mental alertness. It is cleansing to all of the meridians, and can be used effectively when running the meridians as described earlier in this book. It can help open visionary states and it helps establish emotional balance. It is very effective in meditation to determine the emotional blocks or conflicts that are creating health problems. It is most effective when bathed in.

LEMON—Lemon is a fragrance that has been used by many old-time mediums to draw good spirits into the environment. It stimulates clarity of thought, and it has a strong impact upon all mental energies, balancing them. It is a powerful fragrance to use in conjunction with any color therapy. The fragrance plays strongly upon the solar plexus chakra and all conditions associated with it. It stimulates a general release of stress. It relaxes the muscles, and it is cleansing to the lymph system. It has a strong, invigorating effect upon all of the meridians of the body. It can be used in wash water to cleanse it of negativity. It is a strong bactericide and it can stimulate the white corpuscles.

LILAC—A powerful healing fragrance, lilac will balance and align all seven major chakras. It stimulates mental clarity, and it is relaxing to the muscles and to pinched nerves. It has a dynamic influence upon the Governing Meridian, the spinal column, and posture/flexibility. It is also a powerful fragrance to use in opening to the fairy kingdom, especially those who assist in making flower/gem elixirs. It can be used to aid the recall of past lives, especially those impacting upon present health conditions. It stimulates memory and clairvoyance.

MAGNOLIA—This fragrance will stimulate and balance the heart and throat chakras, and thus all conditions and organs associated with them. Anointing the head in meditation will aid in psychic development, especially for finding that which is lost.

MUSK—Musk was used in the Egyptian and Persian traditions to purify the lungs and bloodstream of the spiritual disciple. It awakens the minor chakras of the hands and feet, stimulating self-assurance and confidence. It also has a powerful effect upon the base and spleen chakras and the Conception Meridian. It can arouse the sexual energies. It nourishes the kundalini, and helps to prepare it so that it can impact upon the higher centers.

NARCISSUS—This fragrance can be a "stumper"—a narcotic. It is very relaxing. It is especially effective for those who have difficulty slowing down the wheel of the brain at the end of the day. It relaxes the left hemisphere of the brain, and thus eases insomnia. It is relaxing and soothing.

NUTMEG—As an herb, nutmeg has an hallucinogenic property in its mace (husk). As a fragrance, it stimulates the digestive system. It stimulates the Stomach and Intestinal Meridians. It can ease diarrhetic conditions. It has also been used for treating rheumatism and cold sores.

ORANGE—This fragrance helps us to release the emotional traumas that are creating chronic health problems. It brings clarity and calmness to those times we are overly excited. It can be used to stimulate dreams that clarify fears and doubts. It balances and opens the spleen chakra and it eases all obsessions.

PATCHOULI—Patchouli balances and stimulates the yin meridians of the body. It is balancing to the base and spleen chakras and all conditions associated with them. It aligns the lower two with the heart center, stimulating greater energy for life. Patchouli calms emotions and strife, and it is a fragrance that can be used to ease argumentative conditions and environments. It is known as an aphrodisiac, and this is partly because of its effect upon the feminine energies of the body. It is also good for easing melancholy and overeating.

PENNYROYAL—This fragrance eases nausea, headaches, menstrual cramps, nervous conditions, and skin conditions. It is powerfully protective to the aura, so much so that the negative thoughts and expressions of others are often repelled by it. This fragrance strengthens the spleen and solar plexus chakras. It is beneficial for both the Conception and Governing Meridians.

PEPPERMINT—Mints as herbs are sometimes called the "friends of life." When grown indoors, they purify and energize the environment. Peppermint fragrance cleans the aura of congestion, energy debris we accumulate by contact with outside energies. It is effective in directing the kundalini through the Governing and Conception Meridians. Peppermint fragrance is an antispasmodic. It refreshes, and it stimulates the mind. It helps. us to overcome fatigue. Peppermint is also good for conditions of asthma, bronchitis, and indigestion.

ROSE—Rose is the queen of flowers used by perfumers. In mythology, it was given to the god of silence by Cupid to seal a promise not to reveal the love of Venus and Adonis. Because of this, it was used to wash the ceilings and walls of ancient banquet halls to remind the diners not to reveal what was said in the course of the evening's celebration. As a healing fragrance, it activates and soothes all of the yin meridians, especially the heart. It has a powerful effect upon the heart chakra, and it balances the Governing and Conception Meridians as well. It can also be used to anoint the head to activate the crown chakra to release greater love and healing. It can be used to augment the effects of any modality of healing.

ROSEMARY—This ancient English herb was often used at Christmas time as a token to elves and other friendly spirits. It is extremely powerful as a fragrance to clear the mind of cobwebs. It activates and balances the solar plexus chakra. It stimulates both the brow and crown chakras as well, facilitating inner peace. It brings clarity to the mind and balance to the emotional energies. Burning the dried herb on charcoal in meditation is supposed to open knowledge along the lines desired.

SAGE—Sage is a powerful cleansing and balancing fragrance, whether used as an incense or an oil. It opens up the aura to allow a freer flow of spiritual energy into the physical, while grounding and protecting the physical from imbalance. It awakens psychic faculties and it releases tension stored in the body. It augments the digestive system, and it awakens the heart and solar plexus chakras. It is a good overall tonic to the entire meridian system.

SANDALWOOD—This ancient and powerful fragrance is balancing and stimulating to all of the yin meridians in the body. It is a powerful healing oil, especially when massaged into bruised areas. Individuals who use any form of touch to heal will increase their ability to channel energies through the hands by anointing the palms with a drop of sandalwood oil. It can be used for protection. When mixed with lavender as an incense, it is supposed to facilitate the conjuring of spirits. It stimulates greater concentration in any activity.

THYME—Thyme oil was used in the mid-nineteenth century to help fight typhus. It activates the thymus gland and strengthens the immune system. It can be used to alleviate sleep disorders. It also has a calming effect upon the brow and crown chakras. It quickens the entire healing process. It can be used in meditation for past-life recall and to assist in finding origins of chronic health problems. It is both an expectorant and a diuretic. It strongly affects the Lung Meridian and the Urinary Bladder Meridian.

TUBEROSE—This exotic fragrance once was known as the "mistress of the night." The most virtuous were said to succumb to its influence. It brings peace of mind. As a healing fragrance, it stimulates the crown chakra and aligns it with all of the others. It can be used as a general tonic for the meridians. It also has the effect of strengthening the membranes and tissues. It increases the sensitivity of the neurological system so that you can more easily recognize the effects of emotions on the physical body. It increases inspiration and psychic abilities as well.

VIOLET—This flower is the symbol of modesty and the occult symbol of twilight. Its fragrance, when used in a bath, awakens a general sense of well-being. When rubbed on the stomach, it will alleviate pain in that area. It is balancing to the Stomach Meridian and the Urinary Bladder Meridian. It can be effective for treating the solar plexus imbalances in digestion that create dizziness and headaches. This fragrance and flower is sacred to the fairy queen. Folklore teaches that, with the gathering of the first wild violet in the spring, your dearest wish will be granted.

WINTERGREEN—This is known as the spell-breaking fragrance. It temporarily aligns the subtle energies with the physical, and it is balancing to the spleen, solar plexus, and heart chakras. It helps create greater positiveness in attitude toward dealing with and ridding oneself of health problems.

WISTERIA—Occultists and healers have often used this to stimulate good vibrations in their work. This fragrance activates the heart and throat centers, strengthening the will and the immune system in overcoming an illness. It was often used in wash water prior to gatherings to stimulate positive feelings. In meditation, it is used to help you recognize what you can do regardless of the circumstances. It stimulates all of the meridians, and it calms any strong imbalance within the subtle bodies. It is soothing and stabilizing to the nervous and circulatory systems. It was once known as "poet's ecstasy" because it stimulates greater creative expression. It opens up spiritual perceptions and inspirations. It can be used for higher illumination on any level, including health matters.

afterword

BECOMING THE
RESPONSIBLE HEALER

There are legal, moral, and karmic responsibilities with any healing work. Only medical doctors—not spiritual healers—are au-
thorized to diagnose, prescribe, recommend treatment, or provide a
prognosis. Even water and aspirin are not to be given. You may offer
advice. You may speak of methods that the individual being healed
may wish to explore. You may also provide therapies, but you must
be careful of making claims of their effectiveness.

A healer, especially one working with vibrational techniques, should
never direct energy to another person without his/her permission. It
does not matter whether you know if the person needs it or not. It is an
invasion of privacy. Remember that the illness always provides an opportunity to learn. If we intercede without another's permission, we
may rob them of an opportunity to learn and grow. If you must direct
healing energies, prayers, etc., do so with a qualifier such as "May this
energy be used for the good of _____ according to his/her free will."
In this way, you do not interfere with the karma and energy of the individual inappropriately.

Healing involves treating not only the dis-ease itself, but also the
underlying causes. These causes are primarily fourfold: physical,

psychological, spiritual, and/or karmic. Physical causes are reactions to the physical environment and biological predispositions. Most often it is reflected by the actions of the environment upon the individual. This can be the actual environment or even the thoughts and people we expose ourselves to that can have a negative effect upon the body's energy.

Most ailments stem from the psychological cause. This is the emotional and mental energy effect. Negative emotional states and mental attitudes—whether our own or those we are exposed to—impinge upon our energies, unless we take precautions. They will work themselves into a physical manifestation of dis-ease. Spiritual causes of disease are also metaphysical, like the psychological causes. They can be dis-eases that we bring upon ourselves to force us into higher awareness and powerful new perceptions. They ultimately bring tremendous changes in lifestyles.

Karmic causes are those situations chosen on a soul level to provide a continuing spiral of growth. In actuality, all the other three can be seen as karmic. *Karma* is a Sanskrit word meaning "to do." Anything we do provides opportunity for growth. Thus all of the causes of illness and dis-ease can be placed under the category of karmic. The problem arises when individuals see their illness as payment for past-life experiences.

This is seen in the manner in which many metaphysical healers explain birth defects and handicaps. A person born blind must not have used his/her vision properly or fully in a past life. An individual who is mentally retarded is said to have made fun of such individuals in a past life. We must be very careful in attaching blame in this manner. Blaming past lives for present conditions can often be an excuse not to work to the fullest in the present. Yes, there may be a few cases such as this, but karma is not cruel and punishing. The disease and/or handicap more often than not has its source somewhere in the present.

An old occult axiom teaches us "What can't be cured must be endured." Yes, we may have a predisposition to a weakness, but a healer should help the individual to discover it, even if it is a negative pattern of behavior or a past-life experience, and provide ways of working with it more effectively. There is no dis-ease that cannot be eased in some fashion through holistic techniques, even those that do have their origin in past-life experiences.

Part of the responsibility of a healer is to help the individual find the method or combination of methods that works best for the individual. It involves exploring not just the physical problem, but possible metaphysical causes as well.

The healer must always keep in mind that all healing comes from within. A healer cannot cure anyone through his/her own power. Nor can the healer promise or guarantee a complete cure to anyone. The healer works as a catalyst to stimulate a change in consciousness and a healing change in the energy of the individual. The healer assists the process, but healing is internal to the individual.

To be a healer is to also be an educator. Even in the holistic field, it is not unusual to find people who continue seeking out healings and treatments from others and yet don't change those things that aggravate the conditions. The healer has to be able to recognize this and prevent this from occurring. There are times when it is necessary to say "no" to a treatment.

This may sound very uncompassionate, but the healer does no good if the individual is not learning what needs to be learned. If people come to you for lung problems and yet continue smoking, not exercising, and so forth, they are wasting your time and energy. They are using you as a band-aid remedy for what they do not wish to correct themselves. They are not taking responsibility for their own bodies and energy systems. If we allow them to place us in this position continually, we are no longer serving in a truly healing capacity toward them. Sometimes our separation and withdrawal can be the most compassionate thing we can do for the individual on a soul level.

Working with holistic and vibrational techniques is a way of demonstrating that individuals can truly help themselves. Once they experience this, their whole world takes on a different significance. And this is when healing truly begins to occur. To be a healer does not demand that you yourself have perfect health. This will not occur, as long as you are human. It does not mean that you can neglect yourself either. Many so-called "spiritual" healers neglect their own physical bodies. They overeat, don't exercise, and participate in negative habits, and yet they feel that as long as they are focused in the spiritual, they have no health problems. What it simply means is that the health problems have not surfaced yet, but they will.

Ask yourself some simple questions. "Would I come to me for healing, knowing what my own personal health habits are?" "Would you go to someone for lung treatments who smokes excessively?" This doesn't mean that the healer should be perfect, but the healer should be working to maintain a strong healthy energy on all levels. This includes proper diet, rest, fresh air, and exercise.

Remember that the healer is a channel for energy. He/she will be directing the energy changes, and if his/her own energy is not balanced, what kind of treatment are you truly getting? The healthier you are, the more dynamic and invigorating the energy that flows through you and is directed by you, the more catalytic you become in the life of the person to be healed.

Expand your knowledge of the human energy system, but always treat that knowledge with respect and humility. Hold it in the highest reverence. Use it to ease the sufferings of others and to awaken their own light. Be the healer first of yourself and your own life, then share that light and health with others!

appendix a

THE PUZZLEMENT OF PAIN

It has been said that the only pain that is hard to bear is the pain of others. Everyone's sensitivity to pain varies, but there are many things that can be done holistically to alleviate both acute and chronic pain.

The chart on the following page lists holistic and alternative methods of alleviating pain, as well as traditional methods.

Methods of Pain Intervention

Drug therapy	Surgery
Nerve blocks	Massage
Color therapy	Meditation
Apply heat/cold	Aromatherapy
Music	Nerve stimulation
Sound therapy	Herbology
Acupuncture/pressure	Crystals/gems
Gestalt therapy	Behavior modification
Diet	Relaxation
Biofeedback	Alexander techniques
Movement (dance, yoga, etc.)	Guided imagery
Polarity therapy	Hypnosis
Etheric touch	Psychospiritual
Trager	Psionics/radionics
Rolfing	Aikido
Lomi	Chiropractic iridology
Shiatsu	Others
Homeopathy	

appendix b

LONG-DISTANCE
VIBRATIONAL HEALING

Absentee or long-distance healing can be an effective tool to as-sist an individual. Often people are asked to send prayers and healing to others who are not present. This is something we can en-hance through any of the vibrational techniques described within this book.

The phenomena of long-distance healing are nothing new. It does transcend logical thought processes, but it in no way transcends real-ity. Energy operates on all levels and in many ways not yet under-stood. That which is called psychic energy is the creative life force of all substance. It surrounds us, penetrates us, and is a part of us. It can be controlled and directed, molded and shaped, stored and used. It can be directed by the mind.

Quantum physics has done much to explain the phenomena of psychic energy. It teaches us that all life and energy expressions are connected, and because we are energy, operating on many levels and in many forms, we cannot move without influencing everything in the universe—even if we don't recognize that influence initially. It teaches us that even observation will change ourselves and what is being observed. With higher expressions and focuses of energy, time and space can be transcended. Thus, in long-distance healing we experience the individual in an immediate proximity, regardless of actual time and location.

Vibrational therapies can be used to assist us in concentrating, tuning, and transmitting healing energies. They assist us in achieving a transcendent level of consciousness so that we can employ a more concentrated focus of our healing psychic energies. We develop a controlled use of the mind through vibrational remedies.

For long-distance healing, it is beneficial to have a witness. A *witness* is a term that has come to be associated with the field of radionics. A witness is "anything which will psychically represent the subject" (Charles W. Cosimano. *Psionics 101*. Llewellyn Publications; St. Paul, 1986, p. 82.). A witness can be a photo, a signature, a blood specimen, hair clippings, or anything that can provide a link between you and the person to whom you wish to direct healing vibrations. The witness helps us to link the rational and the intuitive levels of the mind, thus serving to awaken the process of sending energy at a distance.

The witness assists us in creating a thoughtform and in directing it toward the individual more effectively. Through the witness, you are more easily able to establish resonance. It serves to awaken the connection beyond physical levels. It brings the individual "to mind." The healing energy can then be sent regardless of time and space.

Determine ahead of time the kind of vibrational remedies you intend to send. You may wish to use your pendulum to determine this.

1. If you wish to use etheric touch, hold your hands over the witness, and begin your rhythmic breathing. As you do, see and feel the energy streaming out through the witness to the individual to heal and balance. Do this for five to ten minutes.

2. If you are using color therapies, you may do this in several ways:

   • Hold the witness in your hands, and visualize the color(s) healing the individual. Focus on the color energy radiating

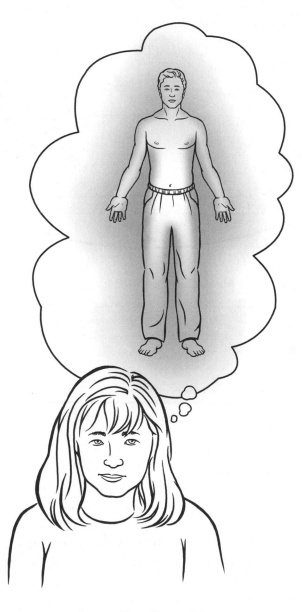

Color Healing from a Distance

As you focus upon the individual, in your mind or through a witness, send colors out to him or her. Use your rhythmic breathing to increase the energy and its projection.

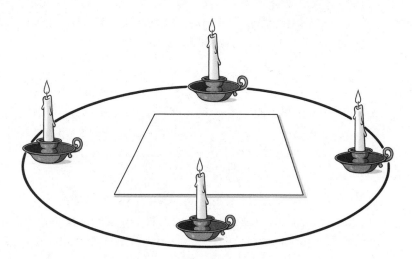

Absent Healing with Candles

Place the witness in the middle of the layout and arrange the color candles accordingly. The color vibrations are then projected and aligned through the witness to the individual. You may wish to use a white taper candle to represent the witness. Simply light it and set it atop the witness. This strengthens the process.

> through you to him/her. Visualize this energy surrounding and permeating their system. See the condition being healed. Perform this for about ten minutes.
>
> • You may wish to project energies through the slide projector. Tape the witness to a piece of white poster board. Then project the colors for each of the seven chakras upon the witness for about thirty seconds each. Then project the primary healing color upon it, and leave it for about ten to fifteen minutes. You can go about your business. This is effective to do at night.
>
> • You may wish to use colored candles as well. Simply place the witness underneath or surrounded by the appropriately colored candle for the healing. As the candle burns, the energy vibration is emitted and it is carried to the per-

son represented by the witness. Do this for fifteen to thirty minutes per day, or more often if needed.

3. You may also use sound and tones. Project the tones at the witness, just as you would if the person were there. This is especially effective in group situations. Place the witness in the center of the group healing circle and tone the appropriate sounds for the condition. Do this for approximately ten minutes.

4. Fragrances and flower and gem elixirs can also be used in long-distance healings. A dab of the fragrance or a drop of the elixir can be applied to the witness periodically throughout the day. The energy pattern of the elixir makes a quantum leap to affect the person that the witness represents.

It is always best to affirm with any healing, especially the long-distance ones, that the healing manifest "for the good of all according to the free will of all." In this manner, the healing occurs in the most beneficial way to the individual's growth. We do not have the right to intrude upon the free will of others, and this is a dynamic way of affecting people in subtle, unnoticed but very real ways.

Do not be afraid to experiment. The extent of the vibrational healing effects is as yet undetermined. Different methods will be necessary for different people. Remember that we each have our own unique energy system, so don't be afraid to adjust the long distance healing accordingly.

appendix c

HEALTH IMBALANCES AND THEIR VIBRATIONAL REMEDIES

The following are guidelines only. They are not prescriptive. They are to help you with your understanding of the effects of vibrational remedies. They will help you find a starting point in working with these subtle therapy forms. They are not designed to replace orthodox medicine. Rather they are to provide you with a means of participating more personally in your own healing process. Do not be afraid to adapt them. Use your own intuition in their application.

In order to fit within the chart, some abbreviations were necessary. In the "Meridian" category, if "Intestines" is listed, this means both the small and the large, unless specifically noted. In the "Sound" category, the first designation is the musical note and the second, the vowel sound(s). In the case of the first, use this tone or a piece of classical or orchestral music written in that key to affect the condition. Under the category of "Elixir" will be listed first the flower elixir and then the gem elixir.

Vibrational Remedies Guidelines

Imbalance	Meridians	Colors	Sounds	Elixirs	Fragrance
Abdominal Cramps	Stomach Intestines	Yellow	E (aw)	Rosemary Citrine	Peppermint
Aches (ear)	Gall Bladder	Turquoise	A (ee)	Turquoise	Eucalyptus
Aches (head)	Bladders (both)	Blue, Yellow	A (ee)	Lavender Fluorite	Lavender
Aches (muscle)	All	Orange	D (oh)	Comfrey Carnelian	Lavender
Aches (tooth)	L. Intestine T. Warmer	Blue	G/A (eh/ee)	Comfrey Turquoise	Clove
Allergies	Lung L. Intestine	Indigo Orange	F/A (ay/ee)	Chamomile Rose Quartz	Gardenia
Alzheimer's	All Governing U. Bladder	Blue, Purple	E/B (aw/ee)	Rosemary Fluorite	Rosemary Violet
Anemia	Pericardium Heart	Red	C	Cinnamon Red stones	
Arthritis	Governing U. Bladder	Violet	Scale	Lilac Amethyst	Lavender Lilac
Asthma	Lung	Blue, Orange	F/G (ay/eh)	Jasmine Turquoise	Eucalyptus Bay
Belching	Stomach L. Intestine	Yellow	E (aw)	Lemon Citrine	Peppermint Lemon
Blood Pressure (high)	Pericardium Heart	Blue, Green	F (ay)	Rose Rose Quartz	Rose Eucalyptus
Blood Pressure (low)	Pericardium Heart	Red, Orange	C/D (oo/oh)	Sage Quartz	Sage Cinnamon
Bones	Governing Kidney	Violet, Lemon	B (ee)	Lavender Amethyst	Lemon Lilac
Bowels	Governing Intestines	Yellow-Orange	D# (oh/aw)	Eucalyptus Carnelian	Eucalyptus Clove

Vibrational Remedies Guidelines (*continued*)

Imbalance	Meridians	Colors	Sounds	Elixirs	Fragrance
Breasts	Conception	Pink	F (ay)	Rose Rose Quartz	Rose Patchouli
Bronchitis	Lung	Blue- Green	F# (ay/eh)	Lilac Turquoise	Bay Eucalyptus
Cancer	All	All but Green	Scale	Lilac Chaparral Amethyst	Lilac Sage Carnation
Colds	Lung L. Intestine Bladders	Red	C/D (oo/oh)	Olive Mustard Quartz	Eucalyptus Bay
Diabetes	Spleen Kidney	Violet	D/B (oh/ee)	Carnelian	Hyacinth
Eyes	Stomach T. Warmer G. Bladder	Indigo, Blue	A (ee)	Pennyroyal Lapis Lazuli	Honeysuckle Rosemary
Fevers	Lung Stomach Bladders	Blue	F/A (ay/ee)	Rosemary Violet Blue Fluorite	Sage Violet Rosemary
Heart	Heart Pericardium	Green, Pink	F (ay)	Rose Jasmine Watermelon Tourmaline	Rose Jasmine
Indigestion	Intestines Stomach Bladders	Yellow	D/E (oh/aw)	Lemon	Lemon
Infection	Bladders Intestines	Violet	B (ee)	Lilac Amethyst	Lilac Frankincense
Influenza	Intestines Stomach	Blues, Violets	G/A/B (eh/ee)	Lilac Amethyst	Lavender Eucalyptus Wisteria
Kidneys	Kidney	Yellow, Orange	D/E (oh, aw)	Gardenia	Lemon

Continued on next page

Vibrational Remedies Guidelines (*continued*)

Imbalance	Meridians	Colors	Sounds	Elixirs	Fragrance
Liver	Liver	Blue, Yellow	E/B (aw/ee)	Carnation Crab Apple	Sage Thyme Pennyroyal
Menstrual	Conception Kidney Spleen U. Bladder	Soft Reds, Blue-green	C/F (oo/ay)	Pennyroyal Hyacinth Pink Tourmaline	Pennyroyal Hyacinth Patchouli
Nausea	Spleen Intestines Liver	Ice Blue	G (eh)	Spearmint	Pennyroyal Nutmeg Wisteria
Nerves	Governing	Blues, Greens	F/G (ay/eh)	Lavender Rose	Lavender Eucalyptus Narcissus
Skin	Lung T. Warmer All	Pinks	Scale	Lilac	Wisteria
Swelling	Depends on Location	Pale and Ice Blues	G/A (eh/ay)	Lavender Quartz	Lavender
Ulcers	Stomach Spleen	Blues, Pale Yellow	D/E (oh, aw)	Peppermint	Peppermint Nutmeg

BIBLIOGRAPHY

General Healing

Becker, Robert, and Gary Selden. *The Body Electric*. New York: William Morrow, 1985.

Donden, Yeshi. *Health Through Balance*. Ithaca: Snow Lions Publishing, 1986.

Hall, Manly P. *Man—Grand Symbol of the Mysteries*. Los Angeles: Philosophical Research Society, 1972.

Hay, Louise L. *You Can Heal Your Life*. New York: Coleman Publishing, 1984.

Judith, Anodea. *Wheels of Life*. St. Paul: Llewellyn Publications, 1988.

Motoyama, Hiroshi. *Theories of the Chakras*. Wheaton: Quest Books, 1981.

Pelletier, Kenneth. *Mind as Healer, Mind as Slayer*. New York: Delacorte and Delta Books, 1977.

Schwarz, Jack. *Human Energy Systems*. New York: E. P. Dutton, 1980.

Steiner, Rudolph. *Health and Illness.* Vol. 1 & 2. New York: Anthroposophic Press, 1983.

Healing through Touch

Brennan, Barbara Ann. *Hands of Light.* New York: Bantam Books, 1988.

Gordon, Richard. *Your Healing Hands.* Berkeley: Wingbow Press, 1984.

Hutton, Bernard J. *Healing Hands.* London: W. H. Allen, 1978.

Krieger, Dolores. *Therapeutic Touch.* Englewood Cliffs: Prentice Hall, 1979.

Seidman, Maruti. *Guide to Polarity Theory.* North Hollywood: Newcastle Publishing, 1986.

Thie, John F. *Touch for Health.* Marina del Rey: DeVorss and Company, 1979.

Yao, Joseph. *Acutherapy.* Libertyville: Acutherapy Seminars, 1984.

Healing through Color

Buckland, Raymond. *Practical Candleburning Rituals.* St. Paul: Llewellyn Publications, 1982.

———. *Practical Color Magic.* St. Paul: Llewellyn Publications, 1984.

Crookall, Robert. *Psychic Breathing.* North Hollywood: Newcastle Publishing, 1985.

MacIvor, Virginia, and Sandra LaForest. *Vibrations.* York Beach: Samuel Weiser, 1979.

Ouseley, S. G. J. *Colour Meditations.* Essex: Fowler & Co., 1944.

Wilson, Annie, and Lilla Bek. *What Colour Are You?* Northamptonshire: Turnstone Press, 1982.

Healing through Sound

Clynes, Manfred. *Music, Mind and Brain*. New York: Plenum Press, 1983.

Crandall, Joanne. *Self-Transformation Through Music*. Wheaton: Theosophical Society, 1986.

David, William. *The Harmonics of Sound, Color and Vibration*. California: DeVorss, 1980.

Hamel, Peter Michael. *Through Music to the Self*. Dorset: Element Books, 1978.

Halpern, Steven. *Tuning the Human Instrument*. California: Spectrum Research, 1978.

———. *Sound Health*. California: Spectrum Research.

Keyes, Laurel. *Toning—The Creative Power of Voice*. California: DeVorss, 1973.

Tame, David. *The Secret Power of Music*. New York: Destiny Books, 1984.

Healing through Flower and Gem Elixirs

FES Society. *Flower Essence Journals*. Nevada City: Gold Circle Publications, 1982.

Galde, Phyllis. *Crystal Healing—The Next Step*. St. Paul: Llewellyn Publications, 1988.

Gurudas. *Flower Essences*. New Mexico: Brotherhood of Life, 1983.

———. *Gem Elixirs and Vibrational Healing*. Boulder: Cassandra Press, 1985.

Richardson, Sarah. *Homeopathy*. New York: Harmony Books, 1988.

Bach Flower Remedies

Barnard, Julian. *Guide to the Bach Flower Remedies*. England: C. W. Daniel, 1979.

Chancellor, Phillip. *Bach Flower Remedies*. New Canaan: Keats Publishing, 1971.

Healing through Fragrance

Beyerl, Paul. *Master Book of Herbalism*. Washington: Phoenix Publishing, 1971.

Cunningham, Scott. *Magical Aromatherapy*. St. Paul: Llewellyn Publications, 1989.

———. *Magical Herbalism*. St. Paul: Llewellyn Publications, 1983.

Fettner, Ann Tucker. *Potpourri, Incense and other Fragrant Concoctions*. New York: Workman Publishing, 1973.

Jackson, Juditch. *The Scentual Touch*. New York: Holt and Comp., 1986.

Lautie, Raymond, and Andre Passebecq. *Aromatherapy*. Northamptonshire: Thorsons Publishing, 1985.

Price, Shirley. *Practical Aromatherapy*. Northamptonshire: Thorsons Publishing, 1983.

INDEX